MARCUS MACFARLANE

FAT IS YOUR FAULT

A successful dieter's perspective on why we're fat, why it's harder than ever to lose weight, and what you can do to share in the happiness of good health.

ATTENTION

UNDER NO CIRCUMSTANCES SHOULD YOU DO OR ATTEMPT ANY OF THE WEIGHT LOSS METHODS OUTLINED IN THIS BOOK WITHOUT FIRST CONSULTING YOUR PERSONAL PHYSICIAN.

I AM NEITHER A DOCTOR NOR A MEDICALLY QUALIFIED PROFESSIONAL.

to your former self

Prologue

Why are you fat? I mean, really, why? Is it simply because you eat too much, or don't get enough exercise? Sure, at the heart of it, that is precisely the reason. But what is it that facilitates and perpetually enables this kind of behavior, and what can we do to fight it? That is the focus of our inquiry.

You've just picked up the last diet book you will ever need to read. You may not realize it yet, but setting down the reading materials is the first step towards realizing your weight loss goals. Just get up and go do it! This volume is a culmination of the knowledge and experiences I have acquired from the short time I've lived here on this earth. Unlike some of the other weight loss readings out there, I'm not going to have you delve into a tome of epic proportions. After all, how are you going to lose weight when you're spending weeks at a time digesting the newest edition of The Atkins Diet? This is the straight-talk, no bullshit diet book. If you are easily offended by some of life's harsh realities, I urge you to read no further. I only promise you one thing. The strategies and guidelines I have put to text here are the same principles that I strive to live by every day. You will lose weight, but only if you commit to keeping an open mind and *stop cheating yourself*. So, tell me, what's it going to be: the red pill, or the blue?

Excellent choice. They say acknowledging the denial of a problem is the first step towards resolving said problem. This phrase is often echoed in the personal struggles of addictive drugs or alcohol abuse, but it is just as relevant a phrase when attributed to unhealthy foods. Unlike other addictions, though, eating is a physiologically compelled behavior required for our very survival. Although essential for human functioning, eating in excess is a serious addiction that can spiral out of control. And, just like any real drug, overeating can cost you a job, a relationship, or your life.

Yes, the commitment necessary to effect real change in one's lifestyle is a difficult and day-to-day process. The same is true of all things in life worth pursuing. I am not here to sugar coat and patronize you into believing that success is expected. Success is earned. Weight loss is not just a subtraction on a bathroom scale; it's a subtraction of food's influence on your life. You will be proud of the weight you lose. That's a promise. Though certain influences try hard to convince us otherwise, there is more to life than Krispy Kremes and KFC. No food exists that *tastes* anywhere near as good as looking good *feels*. Thinness is on an entirely higher plane of consciousness.

There is no secret formula I have hidden up my sleeve for eternal health and youthfulness. Nothing that is documented in this book is anything you can't Google on the Internet or find out from any fitness buff. I can only share with you the methods that have helped me personally attain significant weight loss. My only hope is that at least one strategy I share with you today illuminates that little light bulb above your noggin and inspires in you a new way forward.

I will forewarn you that I am in no regards a medical professional, nor am I licensed to provide medical advice in any form, function, or capacity. You should still consult the wisdom of your personal physician prior to beginning any new diet or lifestyle regimen.

That should be good enough for the lawyers, right? Okay, let's begin.

A Portly Past

"Fatso!"

This is undoubtedly the earliest recollection I have of another person taking shots at my appearance. I was in the 2nd grade. I couldn't have been more than 7 years old. This diatribe, while seemingly trivial in it's individual context, started my life's journey down a long road of vilification and exile from what might be considered a normal childhood.

My hulking size was probably the biggest repellant of most spoken insults. I could crush the life out of those who chose to let loose their real thoughts of me (that is if I could catch them). So instead, most just avoided me entirely. *What purpose does a quiet, overweight fat fuck serve in my life, anyways?* My shyness didn't help much in the way of making friends. The most dreaded words to leave a teacher's mouth were unquestionably, "Okay, class. Find a partner." Group work? I'd rather you go out, socialize, and share my grade later. I don't mind pulling another all-nighter, so long as I don't have to spend 3 hours in a room full of people I don't have much in common with.

I loathed sports, though skipping the summer baseball season was absolutely out of the question in my parent's eyes. I played catcher, as my wide figure was more attuned towards stopping balls than chasing after them. For these couple of months, baseball practice was really the only exercise I got all year. I already weighed north of 160 pounds and was filling out large adult shirts by the time I left elementary school.

I am naturally an introvert, so I took up hobbies that would match such a lifestyle. I joined the school band in the 3rd grade and played alto saxophone through freshman year in high school. I also dabbled a bit in piano and guitar at the time. I was one of the archetypal "band geeks", so to speak. At my school, as long as you took a class in fine arts (i.e. band, drama, chorus), you didn't have to sign up for gym class. That's probably the only reason I stayed with it as long as I did.

My nearly nonexistent social life did have the blessing of allowing me to focus on my academics. While I was no savant, I could cruise through classes without much concentrated effort. I never studied for a test or exam, that is until college threw a good dose of reality my direction. I participated in the middle school's Academic League, a regionally competitive Trivial Pursuit of sorts. We weren't especially awful, but I'm certain that we were never quite ready for primetime Jeopardy. I qualified for the Gila County Spelling Bee when I was in the 6th grade and placed 15th overall. So, if you see any misspellings in this rhetoric, I do apologize. History tells me I should be better than that.

In high school, I delved even more into technological pursuits. I joined the computer club my junior year, having already built my own PC at the age of 13. It seemed like a good fit. *After all, who needs real friends when you have the Internet?* I earned myself an A+ Computer Repair license, the gold standard for Best Buy Geek Squad applicants. I stayed with it and earned a Network+ license the following year.

Things changed a bit for the better socially in my last year of grade school. I shared a study hall during junior year with some members of the school football team, and they convinced me to try out for the team over the summer. My large stature made me an ideal candidate for a lineman position. I didn't end up playing a whole lot. It turns out that walking on to the varsity squad is a lot easier said than done. My first year of football would also be my last, but it did have me associated with some of the more "popular" kids at the school. I was working out before school and practicing after school, football easily becoming the most time-consuming venture of my life to date. The thing was, even as a habitually lazy introvert, I actually quite enjoyed it. For the first time in my life, I actually felt like part of something that matters to people. If you live in small town America, you know high school football is one of the most important social and political forces in the district. While the rest of the school rots into dilapidation, the football team regularly enjoys new uniform sets and funds to support a full coaching staff.

Football was incredibly rough. Going from Kelvin zero to mediocre is no simple task. I was grossly out of shape, and endurance running was something I had never particularly enjoyed. The high impact workouts quickly lead to perpetual strain on my thunderous lower limbs. Shin splints were something I just had to fight through, my ankles slowly crushing into oblivion.

One important lesson I learned was that the sport wasn't about me in any sense. My purpose was to do what I could to help the team as a whole; my ailments were of no concern or consequence. It's a mentality that can't be fully expressed to those who have never been a part of a mission-driven organization. I was thrilled to participate, even as a pawn on the scout team during practice. My only regret when the season ended was that I hadn't joined sooner. So long, Payson High.

The biggest culture shock came when I left home for college. I applied to Arizona State University in 2007, and was fortunate enough to be one of the 95% with a pulse that were accepted for admittance. Never before had I lived on my own accord, bereft of any schedule forced into my hands. *I don't have to take any classes in the morning? Sweet, I'll just fill my afternoons up then. I can sleep until noon everyday! I can go out and drink all night! There's unlimited food at the dining halls? Allow me to take advantage of that.* You always hear about new college students picking up the Freshman 15 when they escape the bounds of their household order. For me, it was the Freshman 50. I lost out on all the physical benefits I had accrued while playing football at home. As for working out everyday? I was lucky to make the trek down to the recreational center once a month.

I quickly regressed into a mess even worse than before. I drank frequently at night, slept all day, and after a few weeks, started missing classes entirely. Being overweight in college *in Arizona* is mortifying, especially when the thousands of girls around you are just so damn fine. The temperature is over 100 degrees well into October, and sweating through fat clothes makes it downright unbearable to be seen in public. It's just my luck that all the perspiration happened to collect in two symmetrical pools right around the breast area, too. Panting around campus with you're dripping tits is, shall we say, less than a great motivating agent to keep showing up to class. And when I did manage to loaf my way over to Psych 101, I became an instant humidifier of stank the moment I sat down. My attitude and environment ultimately got the better of me. I failed my first semester at ASU, straight up. I failed the second one too, but we'll get to that in a minute.

I came into possession of a new car in March of 2008, my pride and joy to this day, a beautiful 2003 Silver BMW M3. This thing is lightning fast, unlike anything the Jeep I had before could ever dream of. Being young and reckless as I was, I pushed the car to the absolute edge when I first got it. The endlessly smooth desert highways beckoned the beast to be unleashed. Whoever owned it before I did must have had the electronic limiter stripped from it, because I hit 170 mph once in the thing and it never showed any sign of holding back.

Unfortunately, the time spent doubling speed limits would soon come to an abrupt end. Easter Sunday, 2008, I decided I would go home and visit my family for the weekend. The normal route from Phoenix to Payson was closed for repair, with the nearest detour being a 3-hour roundabout east through Globe, AZ. Seeing as I had a shiny new ride sitting in the parking garage to whisk me about, I decided to make the journey up home. I enjoyed a nice dinner, after which I returned back to my dorm going down that same detour. Coming from the east into the valley, I had a chance to open up on the US60 freeway in Mesa, a road that is smooth, wide, and dead straight for about 26 miles. This six-lane superhighway appeared to be the perfect proving grounds for a high-speed cruise. Ramping up to about 120 mph, I was just living it up in the carpool lane. The sparse holiday traffic meant I wouldn't have to slow down much from Apache Junction to ASU, but unknowingly blowing past a sheriff's deputy three lanes over would change all that. Only later would I find out that it took the officer a full six miles to catch up with me.

    After crossing six lanes to pull over on the shoulder of the road, I could tell immediately that this cop was clearly not as impressed as I was with the capabilities of the beamer's drivetrain. The deputy drew his 9mm handgun, pointed the business end directly at my face and ordered me "COPS" style out of the vehicle and onto the ground. I was charged with felony evasion of a police officer, a class 5 offense, punishable by up to 3 years in prison. I maintain my innocence to this day, if for no other fact than I had no rational incentive to run. Criminal speeding was a given, no doubt, but felony evasion? No matter, if you've ever been in a legal tussle, you know that the difference means little in the eyes of the law. The officer's report is the word of God, and that's all there is to it. Plead to whatever lesser charges the DA mercifully offers, and move on with your life. Having no prior offenses, I was let off pretty easy. I spent three days downtown in the custody of Sheriff Joe Arpaio. I wore the patented stripes and pink underwear, met the King of the Whites (a sort of tribal thing supposedly), and ate moldy sandwiches. I then proceeded to spend the next year on probation, doing whatever I could to keep my ass from going back to that hellhole.

The worst part of the legal proceedings, more than jail itself, is the unsettling feeling of just not knowing the outcome. *Will the judge be lenient, or am I going to get the book thrown at me?* That stomach-churning stress caused me to pack on even more pounds, as every meal could have been my last as a free man. I started filling out 4XL-sized shirts and became a full-fledged whale by the time sentencing came around in June.

By the age of 18, I'm morbidly obese *and* a convicted felon. Super, my life is really shaping up to be exactly as I had envisioned it. As much as I despise that duplicitous deputy, I thank him for the valuable learning experience he put me through. Looking back now, I believe everyone should be shown what it's like to get arrested at some point in life, just so they can appreciate firsthand the imperfections of the criminal justice system and what "being tough on crime" really entails.

The beauty of being on probation is that it requires you to make positive changes in your life, or else you risk getting hauled away to the slammer. Full-time enrollment in school or employment is mandatory, and I wasn't about to go out and apply at Burger King. I went back to school and started earning actual credits towards my degree, a welcome change to the false start I had the year prior. Staying squeaky clean, I was able to have that felony dropped to a misdemeanor when I was released from probationary custody. What I hadn't been rid of, however, was any of the weight I gained.

With the cloud of the law no longer hanging over my head, I began to run short of excuses for why I perpetuated my spherical existence. That particularly severe impetus of stress was gone, but the stress eating with it somehow missed the memo. In retrospect, I think the true catalyst in change came from seeing how my friends around me were progressing in life. Most by this point were now graduating college (or very near it), and many had steady jobs, girlfriends, or even wives. These are some facets of the high life that I would very much like a taste of. Growing up, I never had the fear of becoming a lazy burnout, because I always did so well in school. But in my early 20s, that's exactly who I saw staring back in the mirror. Success had not come to me as naturally as I felt it would.

Hate and loneliness. Even today, I believe these are the driving forces perpetuating my existence and motivation to improve. I am angry with myself mostly, but I also think of all those who've treated me poorly, shitting on my identity for years and years. They were right all along. *I had no self-control. I was a fat piece of shit that should've crawled into a Hometown Buffet broom closet and died 8 years ago.* I *was* worthless.

I chose instead to prove them wrong; to prove them all to be the stupid, insecure people I knew them all along to be. Prove myself wrong, and tell those little voices in my head to fuck off. For life is but a short experience for us all, and obesity sure closes more doors than just the ones we can't fit through.

My hope, if nothing else, is that this brief synopsis of my past has shown that even unlikely candidates, like myself, can eventually muster up the desire for change that radically alters his or her own future. You are neither "born" skinny, nor can you be "naturally" fat. Until the day they put you in a box, or in an urn on the fireplace mantle, there is hope for you in weight loss. Today is a fresh page in the story of your life. Will it be steeped with the encumbrances of old, or will you author a vibrant and positive change in theme? Join me now as we explore the dynamics of cultural, societal, and socioeconomic influences in shaping our existence, here in America and around the world. I'm Marcus Macfarlane, and you're in The Saturation Room.

1

Family, Friends, and Religion

Evaluating the next direction you take in life can be aided by knowing how it is you got to where you're at in the first place. Why am I fat? What am I doing wrong at this moment in time that I have to change? How do the people around me manage to look like movie stars while they seemingly put forth no effort at all to look that way? The good news is that you too can join the ranks of the aesthetically elite, and the current predicament you find yourself in is not entirely your fault to begin with.

You've probably been told countless times that you're big boned, fluffy, or just not *that* big. When you share with others your struggle with weight loss, people are likely to say, "Who cares if you're fat? You look fine. You carry your weight well." These people are full of shit. Full of it. Those who share a kind word about your ungainly physical appearance are boasting their own self-image by appearing nice. They still think you're a fat mess; they just won't be honest enough to tell you directly. The truth hurts, but lifting that cloud of denial is more crucial to your success than any conceited compliment.

Now, I know I am going to get some flak for this, but one of the key components in your overall being is shaped by your associated faith. Yes, I'm talking about your religion. God wants you to be fat. If you've ever been a member of a religious household, you know that it is an absolute *sin* to waste a scrap of food. *Just think of all those starving children in Africa!* When dinner is served, it is the moral obligation of the family, especially the children, to polish off every little morsel on the serving tray. Seconds, thirds? Sure, why not. It will make you a big, strong, and righteous individual.

What you may not have heard of is what your holy book actually says about overeating. *The body is to be treated as a temple. Gluttony is one of the seven deadly sins.* According to the Word, for all intents and purposes fat people go to hell! Satan can always put to use the plentiful grease of the American obese. For a whole host of logistical reasons, that extra burrito you decided not to stuff your face with was never headed to Sierra Leone in the first place. If you really want to help the starving poor, drop a coin in the red bucket outside Walmart the next time you walk by.

Biblical tides of food serve to instill a sense of humility in children that bad parenting cannot. Those who are fat don't have any platform to judge others upon and are in a sense locked in a prison of their own flesh and blood. It's akin to being caged in the public stocks, where the citizens can hurl atrocities in your direction with no recourse. Congregations are also hurling in your direction the notion that you should blindly follow their deity. Who are you to question God's authority when just about everyone else questions your choice of cheesecake? Humility is a prized characteristic among God's flock, whose singular purpose is to be guided by their enlightened shepherd. Do as you're told then, because judging from your appearance, you have a blatant inability to control your own soul.

Religious leaders also have you believe in a false sense of acceptance about your pudgy self. It is a virtue of god-loving people to be good to thy neighbor, and treat others in a way that you would like yourself to be treated. It's a great creed to live by, but these rules apply to many Christians solely between the hours of 10 and 11AM on Sunday morning. The people who were so caring, friendly, and uplifting to you on Sunday are right back to their spiteful, sinister selves Monday morning. I have no problems at all with the Lord, but his fan clubs are undoubtedly the worst.

Shifting further into the family dynamic, there's an inherent pressure on parents to ensure their kids are well fed. Skinny, small, or underweight kids come off as a sign of neglectful parenting and can be indicative of other underlying problems at home. In response, mothers and fathers stuff their kids silly with unhealthy foods to ward off their nosy peers. *My kids never go to bed hungry, so how could I be seen as anything else than an excellent provider?*

Aother benefit to making a pig out of your offspring: they'll be less likely to supersede the perceived value and worth of their insecure parents. Your dad worked his whole life to be a figure of higher authority than you, and he'll be damned if you look slimmer, make more money, or have more friends than he ever did. If you're a man, he definitely doesn't want your mother to share any more affection with you than she is already withholding from pops.

"Eat up, honey. Don't you want to grow big and strong?" Children are shovel-fed junk food from the get-go in hopes that they will grow up to be anything but skinny and meek. Smaller children are natural targets for bullies and other harassers. Though this may be the norm, giving your child the gift of girth is not helping anyone in today's society.

Gone are the days of unpunished juvenile mischief. If your son or daughter is seen being physically assaulted in any way, you can expect police to swoop in before the words "no tolerance" leave the principal's mouth. The underlying travesty by having an increased police presence is that children who are *verbally* bullied cannot defend themselves *physically* without immediately being subject to reprimand. Your kid may be the one who ends up in juvenile detention, just because he or she couldn't take the abuse anymore and chose to take a stand.

"Get out of the house. Go outside and play!" Not many children today hear these words anymore. It's a foreign concept to kids that are now growing up with Turtle Beach cans strapped to their heads. Helicopter parenting subscribes to the notion that kids are unsafe outside their homes. Every stranger that passes your neighborhood is offering candy to your child from a rusted, windowless van. Kids today are instead socialized through Facebook, Snapchat, and Xbox Live. Personal interaction is dangerous; therefore you are only allowed to communicate anonymously online. Children are fully onboard, too. *What the hell am I going to do outside anyway? Play with a stick? There's not even Wi-Fi out here! I can't share with the world how bored I am right now being out here on the street!* You know what exists outside, rarely used to capacity anymore? Baseball diamonds, soccer fields, and basketball courts.

Traditionally, huge meals have been a staple in the kitchen of hard working families. Three flapjacks, four eggs, six slices of bacon, and a side of biscuits and gravy were essential to fueling up the body for the long day's work ahead. You could eat a 4000-calorie breakfast and expect to burn it off by lunchtime. You might risk fatigue, injury, or just plain hunger out in the field otherwise. In the days before cushy office jobs and robotic automation, hard physical labor was the norm for most folks. Obesity levels were far less than they are today, due in part to these increased activity levels. Neighborhood gyms were few and far between. Your job *was* the gym.

It comes as no surprise then that poor eating habits are passed down from generation to generation. You are far more likely to find an entire family of overweight people rather than one outlying straggler. Just look at the Honey Boo Boo clan. Fat parents, by and large, breed fat kids. A recent study published by the University of Newcastle suggests that children with overweight fathers are four times more likely to be obese by the age of 8. I can personally attest that certain bad habits do indeed roll from the top down. My nuclear family has struggled with our weight for as long as I can remember, and I know for a fact that it didn't start with me demanding Mom and Dad to cook more Lasagna. When you grow up watching those around you scarf down dish after dish made with love, butter, and cheese, it's only natural that you follow suit. In fact, failure to become a member of the clean plate club could be seen as immediate grounds for punishment.

In various cultures around the world, leaving even a scrap of food on your dish is considered an egregious insult to the host. The person serving you the food may automatically assume that you think the food is below your standards and that you are pushing your plate away in a manner of disgust. In other societies, it is common courtesy to leave a small morsel of food on the plate as a show of fullness. If you leave a polished clean plate at the table, the host would take it to mean that their food has insufficiently filled your appetite. You may get shot a dirty look, or you may find your plate being piled on with extra helpings.

As a kid, I remember how the amount I ate in one sitting served as a degenerative source of pride. I would strive to eat a Super Size McNugget meal every time I went to McDonalds, because I believed it was the coolest thing to do. I didn't want to be the scrawny kid who was 8 inches shorter than me, primed to be knocked over by the next brief gust of wind. Even in high school, I would order six tacos and a double bacon cheeseburger with fries at Jack in the Box, stuffing myself every time I ate until I could eat no more. The athletes at school all seemed to eat just as much, why couldn't I? Bigger is better, I thought. Only later did I realize that "bigger" is just bigger.

Self-control is not a concept most overweight people are familiar with. In fact, table manners may be the only form of self-control your family practices on a regular basis. *Don't eat until everyone has sat at the table and has a plate in front of them. Never eat until you've thanked your lord and savior for putting that KFC on the table. Don't drink until you've clinked glasses with the other members of your party in an appropriate toast.* The one that can really affect you proportionately, however, is *the rule to wait for everyone to be done eating before you excuse yourself from the table.* You may have finished your coconut shrimp five minutes into the dinner service, but Grandma is going to need the better part of a half hour. No phones allowed at the table, so browsing cat pictures on Reddit will just have to wait.

Sitting there, straight as a board, no elbows on the

table, you pretend to be engaged in your family's stories of their friends and distant relatives, many of whom you've never met. As you're listening to the intimate medical details of your aunt's cousin's appendicitis, you can't help but smile and stare blankly at the empty dish before you, stabbing at hollowed potato skins with your butter knife. Boredom has set in on levels you thought were reserved only for 3rd period English, so eating more inevitably becomes your only reprieve. "Pass the biscuits, please," you mutter in surrender.

Speaking of family gatherings, there's no shame is gaining an extra 10 pounds when the holidays come around. You'll be that much further ahead for swimsuit season next year if you resist the urge, though. Thanksgiving marks the annual start date for letting go, throwing sound advice to the wind, and gobbling down the cobbler. For kids, it starts even earlier at Halloween. Crafty youngsters can procure a month's worth of sweets in one night if they canvass the right neighborhoods. Holidays are a free pass, and many in your family are likely to give into temptation right alongside you. Colder weather is setting in, and most people look bulky anyhow with the added layers they're wearing around town.

Holidays are often a stressful period in our lives, and one of the main combatants of familial anxiety packages itself in the form of alcohol and party platters. You may find it unbearably tempting to dive into the cheese and cracker plate while your aunt elucidates, in excruciatingly fine detail, every sore, toothache, and broken nail plaguing your extended family. *Oh, your medical insurance denied that wart removal last month? I give two shits of a flying fuck! Please, continue your story while I smile and drown myself in eggnog.*

It's one thing to try and hold back at the family reunion, but your greatest enemy of weight loss if often the person whom you love and trust the most. In fact, your wife or girlfriend can be the very Satan of Supper. No longer living the life of a scrounging bachelor, your significant other often tries to get to your heart through your digestive tract. It can be the greatest feeling in the world to have a medium rare steak and a baked potato waiting for you when you get home from a long shift at work. If you're lucky enough to snag a lady who whips up a miracle every meal, most would say you've got yourself a bona fide keeper. Multiply this by five weekdays, add in dinner dates on the weekend, and before long you're living in a hog's heaven.

As the months and years progress, that hog heaven can progressively devolve into hell's kitchen. You find yourself rarely skipping meals anymore, a far easier feat as a bachelor.

If one of you is hungry, chances are that the other is going to pony up and eat right along with you. You can't just settle for a bowl of Cheerios in the morning, either. You have to cook every meal like you mean it. Bacon and eggs and spaghetti and meatballs stir romantic interests far more than a microwaved Lean Pocket. Feast like a man, or risk being thought of as less than.

The masculinity of your diet can rapidly lead to weight gain, a devious fantasy realized by both partners in a relationship. Growing old and fat together is what most couples dream of, yet really this just entails making your partner as unattractive to the competition as possible. Fat lovers are seen as more loyal lovers, but not by choice. Your options for extramarital affairs dwindle significantly when you let yourself go. Past flames are less likely to rekindle when your ex sees what effects gravity and Gouda have had on their former lover's physical appearance. Domestic power, relative to your spouse, can shift greatly depending on your current waist measurement. It is best that you meet or exceed the increasingly lowered standards of your partner, if not but for your own sake.

Stuffing each other's faces isn't always a subconscious act of subterfuge either. Some even get off on it. Known as "feeders," these special kinds of people plug their partners full of sweets to quench their own sexual fetishes. *Oh yeah, baby, the slurping, the chewing, and the farting really gets me going!* Watch out for the warning signs. If you're regularly enjoying cake and ice cream in bed, and she's just lying there next to you biting her lip, you may have a feeder on your hands. If she gets cold and distant anytime you deny her pecan pie, you might want to get the hell out of there. If your happiness is truly important to your lover, he or she should not be digging you a sugary grave. A mildly relevant thought just crossed my mind. If you haven't seen it yet, I highly recommend the movie *Feed* for an obscene example of what a feeder is capable of. Actually I don't *recommend* it, but you or your feeder girlfriend might want to watch it. It's like a drug addict watching *Requiem for a Dream*. It may just scare you straight.

    This sick sabotage extends not only to your significant other, but likely to any children you share together. Parents are naturally afraid of their children growing up, hating them, and moving away. This happens most when kids find a girlfriend/boyfriend they like, a good job, or a college out-of-state. Children are treated like property to many, and parents will be damned if you leave to pursue your own life's vision. Momma's boys and Daddy's girls strive to please their parents at their own expense, sacrificing their own happiness to support a parent's wishes. More unruly offspring will have to be coerced into obedience. Fattening up the kids will keep them loyal to you, as nobody else their age will want to be associated with them. The overly attached parent is sheltering their children by doing this, rather than preparing them for the harsh realities of the real world. Okay, so your fat kid can't play dangerous sports or be duped into relationships with shallow partners. Instead, they play in the band and live in the World of Warcraft as a keyboard killer. What an upside!

A wise man once said, "Tell me the company you keep, and I'll tell you who you are." Your character, personality, and behavioral patterns are primarily a weighted average of the people whom you share time with. If you grew up in suburbia and went to private school, you will probably end up as an Ivy League power player hailing from a great fraternity of compatriots with similar upbringings. On the flip side, someone growing up in a Section 8 apartment in an inner city community goes through the public school system. He or she is likely to be exposed to a criminal underground with drug dealing gangs and financial insecurity. Many children born into these circumstances are lucky to attend community college or even graduate high school. I'm not here to lament about the economic disparity we see across geographic regions in America. There are many who will rise from rags to riches, and many from the top who crumble into destitution.

More importantly than any financial or educational similarities you might share with your friends is what you share as you break bread. I'm sure you are familiar with the various cliques that form as you progress through school and into the real world. Most social clubs are wrought with inside jokes and an inflated sense of esteem, but it provides members with that much-needed sense of purpose or belonging. The gamers, the band geeks, the drama queens, and the jocks all hang together, and each group thinks their club is the bee's knees. There's a reason that those involved with sports tend to be the more popular and in shape bunch. Their interests revolve around weight training, aerobic activity, and cheerleaders. Popular chatter centers around supplements, protein shakes, and the bench press. The A/V club throwing LAN parties on weekends brags about their K/D ratios and have shopping lists consisting of Mountain Dew, Doritos, and hydroponic weed.

Fat people are more likely to hang out with friends who share their skewed views on dieting and health in general. Going out to Chipotle for lunch three times a week is socially acceptable when your friends are shoveling in the same barbacoa burritos. You can even pitch in and share the bottle of Chipotlaway for later, if you catch my drift. In high school, I used to frequent the local Chinese buffet at least twice a week. But since I had likeminded friends who were eager to join in, I didn't see any tangible backlash for loading up on a third plate of crab puffs and chicken lo mien.

Friends have their own hidden agenda at play when choosing to surround themselves with your superfluous presence. It looks good on them, speaking volumes to their own character. For one, it's great to have a personal bodyguard hanging around. You make your friends look important, like they require that added layer of protection. On an added note, girls think your friends are kind-hearted people for not being judgmental of your appearance. Women think this translates to how their new boy toy will treat them, not being overly critical of *their* looks. Good on them, tonight your friends got laid! Bad on you, tonight you're stuck with the DUFF of the girls or (the majority of the time) strapped in for a long night on PornHub.

One way friends can undermine your personal weight loss efforts is to brag about just how much junk food they consume. "Ugh, I can't eat anymore. I just finished a whole pizza at lunch." You may think that this isn't possible. *How can you look so good after eating all that crap!* The solution resides in the metabolism of your compadres. Likely, that pizza is the only misstep they've had all week in straying from their usually well-balanced diet. Furthermore, they probably have been working out at the gym all week just to enjoy that one whole pie. However, just knowing that your slender friends can eat tons of food without regret hurts your obese mindset. You feel bad that you can't eat the same and look that good, but you go back to scarfing down that same food regardless to fill that pit of shame.

Don't even think about touching that salad, or you may find yourself further subjugated to the chides of your fellow peers. It may seem paradoxical, but trying to change your eating habits to look and feel better is frowned upon by many. "You've been eating cheeseburgers your whole life, why on earth would you have a salad for lunch?" Screw these people. You have to start somewhere, but prepare for the criticism to continue unless you hold strong in your lifestyle change. One salad at noon to offset a three-egg omelet and a porterhouse steak is not going to further your efforts in the slightest. This is what your friends get off on; the fact that they know you'll be back to old habits later. Stick to cutting back for a few weeks, though, and you're going to be savoring that last laugh for yourself. Inside they'll be quietly petrified, suddenly gauging a higher awareness of their own dieting follies.

A common expression many comedians are familiar with is the phrase "comedy is born of misery." Indeed, a healthy percentage of the stand-up acts you see at local improvs or on television began their careers medicating their own personal anguish with humor. These performers are laughing on the outside, crying on the inside. You often hear of the "funny fat guy", the member of a social group whose singular purpose is to entertain others with a deft combination of sly undertones and witty quips. Often possessing little or no other applicable life skills in comparison to their athletic peers, the gift of making others split their seams laughing is a trait that few others execute well. Already designated an easy target to lash out anger upon, the funny fat guy cements his place in friendship by allowing his existence to serve as a punching bag to the beautifully cursed. Some of the more well-known examples include Ralphie May, Gabriel Iglesias, John Candy, and Chris Farley. Have you ever listened to one of their audiotapes? I sure haven't. Much of the best material from these comics stems from incorporating their prominent physical attributes into the act. *Fat guy in a little coat! I'm not fat, I'm fluffy!* The audience is crying in tears, sure. But late at night, long after the curtains have closed, these comedians are in dark hotel rooms wallowing in shame. The very success of the funny fat guy is correlated with his waist size, perpetuating a miserable cycle many are reluctant to break. Losing 100, or even 200 pounds would be a great personal achievement. However, the professional and financial implications may leave a promising career hanging out to dry.

Unless you can grind a living out of people laughing at your expense, losing weight can be a matter of personal survival. Life is a dog-eat-dog game. There are no participation trophies in the game of life. Everything worth achieving involves competition, where the weak inevitably fade into nothingness. You will always be fighting for jobs, status, or just about anything else you can imagine. The niceties your so-called "friends" share with you are subversive attempts to train you to be accepting of your existence in its current state. They don't want you to lose the weight. If that happened, all of a sudden you'd evolve from benign comedic relief into a full-blown threat to their positional power.

This is something I experienced as I lost the weight. People I have known for years became a lot more aggressive and visceral in their demeanor, especially when their girlfriends started checking me out. Be wary, as you lose weight this is likely to happen to you. Your well-being may come at the expense of the happiness and contentment of others. *So be it.* In money management, the first rule is to *pay yourself first*. In personal health, you have to *love yourself first*. In effect, you are flipping the tables from being the oppressed to being the oppressor. Those who criticized your life's choices in the past are suddenly going to turn and question their own decisions, and that is when you win.

2

The Working Environment

Stress in the workplace is a perk issued when you start working at most offices. Stress is a motivator. It serves as a constant reminder of the expectations and deadlines that you are required to meet. A job that is vacant of stress is a job without fear of repercussion, and the finished work often suffers as a result. It is the primary objective of the manager, supervisor, or boss in general to make sure that you, the employee, are earning every cent of your paycheck.

The introduction of stress, while fruitful, does come with its share of unintended consequences. Employees in fast-paced work environments are drowning in anxiety on a daily basis. Bosses are a stick in the mud, and the clients are even worse. Every day feels like a fight for survival, because your livelihood is often hanging on by a mere thread. Bills at home need to be paid, and one bad day at the office could have you piling your things into a cardboard box.

Living life one day at a time is a dream for many, but it

is not the wisest way to approach life. If today could be my last day, I might as well enjoy what employed time I have left and celebrate. *Donuts for breakfast? Sure, why not? Better grab a dozen for the coworkers too. I'll have just one here in the car while I wait in traffic. Scratch that thought, my colleagues can fight over a half-dozen. My half hour lunch break started five minutes ago? Looks like I'm going to have Chicken McNuggets for the third time this week. The vending machine down the hall has eaten enough of my 401k as is.*

Comfort foods are a great distraction to the chaos of the workplace. If it's not donuts for breakfast, it's a birthday cake for lunch. You could have fifty slices of birthday cake a year if you work in a big firm. Treats are the perfect distraction for a team at work, especially for boosting morale. There's nothing quite like a sugar high to get over a case of the Mondays. These sugary foods make you feel special, if only for a moment, in an environment where others are backstabbing or stomping on your throat.

If eating to quell stress isn't your only impetus, eating to stifle boredom is another many of us can relate to. Work sucks. If you're not plugging away at TPS reports, then you're listening to eight different bosses reprimand you for failing to put a cover sheet on them. *It's that time of year again for the* sexual harassment seminar? How about I sexually harass this Reese's peanut butter cup instead? I already took a nap earlier while my supervisor was in a staff meeting.*

Okay, so what if I prepare healthy meals at home and bring my own lunch to work? This may be your best bet in sidestepping the landmines around you. If you keep a salad in the break room, you're already miles ahead of the competition. Be warned though, the fridge also harbors some of the easiest game in the building. *Why would I eat that turkey wrap I made this morning when I can hijack Sally's leftover linguine? If only my wife knew how to cook like her.* My stomach cares little about you slapping your name on the Tupperware container. *You're not going to drink that entire 2-liter of Dr. Pepper either, so I may as well snag a glass before it goes flat.*

The break room isn't the only trap to avoid at your job either. Clientele subscribing to high profile firms expect to be pampered when unloading a fortune into the company coffers. Some of the most important deals in business are made as your taking your clients out for a fancy evening at the city's premier steakhouse. Even if you insist on ordering a salad every time you're out schmoozing industry titans, good luck resisting the urge to down the loaf of free bread when it comes to talking brass tacks.

As an employee whose job requires you to interact with customers on a daily basis, personal appearance can make all the difference. Your boss wants representatives of the company to project a lean, fit image to the public. It becomes very difficult for customers to buy into your sales pitch when you make yourself hard on the eyes. When people see that you have no control over your weight, what would make them think they should give you control over their finances?

The opposite can be true if you're buried in a cubicle on a 3rd floor office. Since clients are likely to never come face to face with your "behind the scenes" position at the corporation, you are free to eat as much as your swivel chair can support. If you possess a unique technical skill or are a "rock star" in your position, bosses and colleagues will often attempt to sabotage you in any number of ways. The reason for this is to mitigate your career aspirations, be unemployable to other companies, but give management just enough reason to keep you around. Good luck trying to snag a larger salary when the competitor's headhunter come knocking on your door, especially when you're breathing through your mouth and sweating from your armpits during the interview.

3

Media and Advertising

Television is perhaps the greatest tool of the powers that be use to influence the food decisions you make. It's hard to go more than 10 minutes watching your favorite shows before once again, delicious food appears before your eyes. Most often, you will be presented with the offerings of the latest fast food fare in your area. Cheeseburgers, tacos, French fries, chicken nuggets; the list goes on and on. Corporate fast food has a mission to churn an insatiable desire for artery blocking, blood pressure raising meals out of its customers.

The goal of the fast food industry is to get you in the door for your very next meal. "Hurry in today!" or "See you tomorrow!" are clever sign-off phrases aimed to get you through the double doors for dinner. Their sly taglines are designed to make you feel like you're missing out on an experience that only their restaurants can provide, right this minute. If you don't get in the car immediately and head to the drive thru, there's a chance that you'll miss out on this limited-time offer and have to settle for the same old, same old from their competitors. *What a drag!*

Limited-time only promotions are a great marketing strategy to boost sales during seasonal lulls. For Catholics who swear off meat during the period of lent, unlimited Fish Fry Fridays draw in enormous crowds that see bottomless cod as a challenge accepted. McDonald's Filet-o-Fish and the release of Fish McBites suggests even Ronald himself is clamoring for that sanctimonious skrill. Restaurants don't just target Bible thumpers, either. Endless shrimp and pancakes, paired with limitless soup, salad, and pasta strikes a spiritual chord with the American public, promising customers that they'll never see the whites of their plates.

It's not just the quantity of food that entices customers. Many simply wish to try something new, anything to distract them from Mom's inedible meatloaf. The McRib arrives but once a year, but for many it becomes a staple of their daily menu for the period it's available. *It's here, right now, so come stuff your face before it disappears!* Who cares if it's a calorie bomb? You'll just have to inhale enough pressed ribs to hold you over until they come around this time next year.

And don't be a sissy, grab that extra large Mountain Dew from Taco Bell on your next visit. *Salad? pfffttt. Be a man, I don't want to see you leave that drive-thru without a XXL Chalupa, Nachos BellGrande, and Cinnamon Twists clenched firmly in hand.* You see, restaurants promote the unhealthiest items on their menus because those items are typically their bestsellers. Furthermore, the specialty grease-laden foods are the most profitable. *Is a Baconator really worth four times the price of a Junior Bacon Cheeseburger?*

When was the last time you saw a McDonald's ad for a Southwest Chicken Salad, or any salad for that matter? *Wait, Marcus! But wait! What about those apple packets they put in Happy Meals now?* Those ads were plastered on TV everywhere. Children now eat healthy at McDonald's! *Oh, really?* What the company reps fail to advertise is that the apples are simply thrown in with the standard McNuggets and Fries, not to mention many have enjoyed an extra dose of listeria with that fresh fruit. Can you remember a time when a Happy Meal left on a smile on your face? I'd say it's more like a queasy kick in the gut. In business, this strategy is known as *societal marketing*. In other words, your company promotes a leaner, greener society without actually doing much to contribute. *Think of Toyota and how all those cute little Prius cars are saving the environment!* Get real, people. These media pushes are used to much less humanitarian ends: brand reputation and boosting sales of their planet-killing Camrys.

Some businesses realize that their products are less than lean, yet they push a message to the masses as if they are. You've often heard the words "organic," "free range," or "non-GMO" tossed around. Chipotle is one of these restaurants that pride themselves on serving burritos sourced from only the most natural and humane ingredients. *Great, the little pigs get to go outside once in awhile. Whoop dee friggin' doo! Those pigs probably spend more time outdoors than you do!* That doesn't change the bottom line. The mass of the burrito they're serving is even bigger than what you'd find at a Taco Bell, and soon your figure will match that.

Other "fast casual" restaurants are guilty of the same moral turpitude. Gourmet sandwich joints like Panera Bread or Wildflower Bread Company trick you into thinking better quality transmutes into better health. A 1% decline in your risk of developing liver cancer 30 years from now is not going to overshadow the massive uptick in your chance of getting heart disease in the same period. All things considered, calories are calories. We'll touch more on that a bit later.

Some restaurants have cast shame to the wayside and actively promote the abominable effects of their menus. One company that comes to mind is the Heart Attack Grille, a burger joint perhaps best known for its Quadruple-Bypass burger. Yes, their burgers are named after heart operations. Clocking in at several thousand calories apiece, one burger at the Heart Attack Grille could sustain a healthy adult for nearly a full week! But don't forget about the unlimited Flatliner Fries on the side. Deep fried in 100% pure lard, these french fries are "worth dying for!" Dressed up in hospital gowns and waited on by "nurses," patrons at the Grille are treated more like terminal patients than mere porkers. Serious eaters at the Heart Attack Grille look to the menu as a challenge, and all customers exceeding 350 lbs. eat **free of charge**. Much to no one's surprise, several spokesmen and loyal patrons of this establishment have died in recent years.

Jared Fogle (prior to the whole "diddlin' kids" thing) showed the world that shedding pounds was as easy as walking in to your local Subway restaurant. Marching downtown for a six-inch sub every day, the former fireman lost an enormous amount of weight and caught the eye of Subway when a former roommate of Fogle's wrote an article to the school paper about how unrecognizable his friend had become. Jared soon became an international sensation and the prime spokesperson for a sandwich shop that was, at the time, skeptical of promoting informal health claims about its food.

Subway sales doubled to $8.2 billion when Jared took the reigns at the helm of Subway marketing. He was so valuable to the company that in 2005 the company took a 10% hit to revenue when Jared chose to take a hiatus. The people of America desperately want to share in the success story of an average guy who lost weight by eating sandwiches. The problem with this logic is that many people are fooled into believing that a Philly cheesesteak or a chicken, bacon, ranch sub is going to magically melt the fat away, when quite the opposite is true. Eating an entire footlong of anything other than a turkey or veggie sub is going to set you back miles in your thin quest. Jared ate a 6" sub at a time, and never did he ask for any mayonnaise, ranch, or any other calorie-chocked cream sauce. In actuality, you're about as likely to find a healthy meal at Subway as you are at McDonalds. It's all about the choices of ingredients you select, and there's a whole load of traps on the other side of that sneeze guard. Who's to mind any sense like that, though, when the American Heart Association just came in and endorsed Subway as the first ever restaurant to have a "heart-approved menu"? At least Subway's business heart is in the right place now. The best reality check they have going for them has got to be their new slogan, "Train hard. Eat Fresh." Athletes eat at Subway to fuel up for the big game, and they exercise consistently to stay in peak shape. That's the more true-to-life message that should be transmitted.

If power walking like Jared down to the local eatery isn't your cup of tea, how about ordering food from the comfort of your couch instead? Pizzas, sandwiches, and Chinese delivery are about as convenient as it gets when it comes to snagging good eats. The Internet has even paved the way for online ordering, further eliminating the hassle of picking up one's phone. *Have you seen the Dominos pizza tracker? Talk about one of the greatest innovations of the 21st century!*

Take-out has revolutionized many other chain restaurants as well. No longer do you have to wait an hour for lousy service at the Olive Garden. Simply order ahead, roll up your Suburban to the designated parking space, and someone will greet you in the lot with dinner for four.

I could rant on the specifics of each and every restaurant you've visited in your lifetime, but at least now you have been exposed to some of the fraudulent activities restaurants are fronting on the good citizens of this nation. Should you manage to repress the enticing allure of Doritos Locos Tacos from your train of thought, there remains but one thing left to accomplish. You really have to turn off the tube and get off that couch! How many overweight people have told you they don't own a television? I know I haven't met any. TV is the archenemy of motivation. While you lose yourself in the vicarious living of the characters on screen, your body continues to atrophy an equal and reactive amount.

- **Screen Actor's Gout**

Television and movie stars share one common characteristic: they're hot. Actors and actresses are, by and large, ideal specimens of human beings. Their unattainable looks are so superior to those of the general public that networks shell out billions every year to keep them on screen. *Why don't they make more TV shows with average looking people?* Simple. They don't normally score well in the ratings. People get disinterested very quickly when they see normal looking folk acting out for the cameras. They want to see every character shown in picture perfect fashion, because who really wants to see how actual detectives or doctors look like? This reality of screen actors is both appeasing and depressing to the viewers. We don't want our heroes to be slobs, but simultaneously we've come to the sorrowful conclusion that we'll never be as cool or as good looking as they are. This sense of futility can lead us to say "Fuck it, might as well finish off the Haagen Daaz tonight."

When shows depict obese characters, they are principally slotted in supporting roles. Often the only reason they exist at all is to provide comic relief. To quote *The Hangover*, "It's funny because he's fat." These representations reinforce today's stigma of taking out abuse on fluffy outcasts. It's okay to make fun of them; they're different from us. It's no less a discriminatory practice than prejudicing against people of different colors, gender, or sexual orientation. What's unique about the topic of obesity, though, is that overweight people have the ability to alter their appearance. The world is not going to get any nicer or reform its general perspective of you, regardless of your efforts. If you're waiting on the world to change (cue song), you're going to be waiting until your dying breath. We only have the ability to change the way we feel and look about ourselves.

The shows that do feature normal or overweight "real" Americans are typically those the media dub as "train wreck TV." Jerry Springer, Maury, and Steve Wilkos all want you to feel better about yourselves as you watch. It's so easy to point fingers at the screen and judge the exploits of the guests on their shows. *As long as I'm not the father, I must be doing something right with my life! I'm a good person because I don't smoke crack or hit my wife. Why bother doing something meaningful about my weight? Did you see that beluga transsexual they had on earlier? I'm miles ahead of him/her in the fitness category already.*

    Having become a popular trend in television, train wreck TV envelops much of the primetime lineup on a whole slew of cable networks. Every program on TLC features a person or family of a peculiar subset put forth for your gawking pleasure. Little people, big people, Muslim people, Amish people, psychic people, and even a show about a guy with a 132-lb scrotum are just a few of the scholarly programs you'll find on "The Learning Channel." "History" Channel and "Discovery" Channel are offloading the same brand of garbage week after week. I've learned how to negotiate with a pawnbroker and make moonshine in the Appalachian Mountains, but I still know jack shit about the Spanish Inquisition.

    Then there's *The Biggest Loser*, the boot camp competitive show where hostess Jillian Michaels screams at her grotesquely obese contestants until they lose half their weight (and their hearing). The home they live in abounds with tantalizing sweets and delectables crying out for their consumption. The weak succumb to temptation. The strong persevere and some even change their lifestyles for the better after the show ends, a commendable feat indeed. Many look to *The Biggest Loser* for pointers on losing weight themselves, but the show features such a rigorous regimen that it is nothing short of intimidating for most viewers. Yes, during the span of a couple of months, the people on *The Biggest Loser* are forced to take such drastic measures that they do succeed in the short-term. But life is long for the rest of us beyond the small screen, and good dieting isn't normally akin to basic military training. If you feel like you need the guidance of these experts because you can't motivate yourself, I wouldn't recommend pigging out in hopes of auditioning for the next season. As soon as these people get off the elliptical machine and out of the limelight, more than half fall back into their previous routines.

It's very rare for overweight folks to reach the upper echelons of stardom and fame. Take a look at the hot items in pop music today. You've probably heard the songs of Adele or Meghan Trainor. These women have the pipes of an angel, yet you won't find these talented artists plastered on every magazine and Covergirl billboard out there. While their songs may hit #1 on iTunes for weeks at a time, the fact is their vocal acumen is merely compensating for their severe lack of physical talent. Adele is worth only a fraction of what other pop stars like Lady Gaga, Christina Aguilera, or Beyoncé are worth, and that's because she'll never be on the cover of Maxim or listed as People's "Sexiest Woman Alive".

This industry ceiling applies for men as well. You won't see a shirtless John Goodman advertising Chanel No. 5 in a seductive black and white TV commercial. Unfortunately, for an actor of his caliber, his weight has likely precluded him from securing an A+ role on stage and screen. Jonah Hill, the Oscar-worthy thespian that has transcended the funny fat guy archetype, will continue to play second fiddle to the Leo DiCaprios of the world. It's just too difficult to remain culturally relevant when the only times a person sees you on screen are in a 90-minute movie or a half hour sitcom.

Sure, there are a few programs on major networks that feature a Rubenesque leading man or woman. *Roseanne, The King of Queens, Mike & Molly,* and others prove that not only supermodels get to hog the tube time. However, it isn't long before you notice that these shows' major "shtick" is to make fun of the fat actors for being fat. It's physical comedy in all its existential glory. Tell me: is that something you really want to relate to in a character?

- **Food Porn**

And don't even get me started with the Food network. I doubt anyone can resist the trance state this network hypnotizes us into. The pornographic close-ups of the best meals around the world are jaw-droppingly infatuating. It's the absolute worst channel to watch when eating or when full, but at a time when you're craving a snack? It's about to be Epic Meal Time up in this house! Unless you're working on a remedy for your severe lack of skill in edible meal preparation, the Food and Travel channels both should be blocked from your cable box.

One star of the Food Network has pushed so much filth onto her viewers that it has resulted in the shortcomings of her own personal health. Paula Dean, the Queen of Southern cuisine, has sampled so many of her own mouthwatering dishes that she now has adult onset diabetes. *Who would have thought that emptying the butter, sugar, and cheese reserves into every one of her recipes would foreshadow any negative health effects at all?* Never one to let a food crisis go to waste, she then advocated a more balanced approach to southern hospitality and has even lost a few pounds. Soon thereafter she decided to have a morally questionable dinner party, and now she's probably back to her old ways. The circle of life continues.

I tell you to block the food channels, because removing these succulent temptations from your life involves limiting your daily impressions of unworldly eats. Instead, you must program your own vision of a healthy, home-prepared meal. If you know of any alcoholics in your life trying to "stay on the wagon," then you know how this works. You're having a dinner party this weekend and all of your friends are invited. Cocktails start around 4 o'clock. One of your good friends just got his 3rd DUI last month, and being the good friend that you are, offer to pick him up for the occasion. His response is, "No, thanks. I don't want to be around all that alcohol."

It makes sense. If I'm going to be in the presence of others downing away at the bottle of Jack, I'm going to be taking shots right there with you. On TV, Adam Richman is sitting right across the table from you devouring an entire pizza in the course of a 30-minute show. When it comes time to hit the fridge during the commercial break, the leftover egg white quiche I'm staring at is just not going to cut it. Have you ever made a healthy, gourmet meal in 30 minutes? Unless you have your own personal studio techs running to buy groceries, measuring ingredients into perfectly portioned dishes on your counter every time, I'd venture to say *no*. Rachael Ray, stop making it look so easy for the rest of us. McDonald's is right around the corner from my house. That's a 10-minute meal round trip.

    The road to hell is paved with good intentions. Sure, you could run into the store to grab a salad for about the same amount of time, but the mind is sure to drift quickly when the billboards on the way there start pelting you with those salacious seven-foot-tall Big Macs. *Enlarged to show texture, my ass!* Those bright, colorful signs with catchy taglines are guiding your vehicle directly to the nearest drive thru window. As you pull into the parking lot, prepare to be further inundated with window-sized posters showcasing the latest and greatest offerings the restaurant has to serve. *Five chicken nuggets for a buck? Better give me a box of 20. You're damn right I want sauce with that! Stuff that bag with ranch dressing, because a dry McNugget isn't worth its weight in bird paste.*

- **Pubs and Bars**

    If you're in no hurry to get home after a shift, your local brewery can serve as the ultimate oasis from the flaring tempers of marital tension. Happy hour is a pub promotion pastime, luring many patrons through their doors following a hard day's work. The beer specials end at 6 PM, but you're not relinquishing the barstool for another eight rounds. The game just finished the first quarter, and you've got $100 on the spread. Your ass is going nowhere. You remind yourself that you're a lightweight and need to get to bed early. Well, that responsible mindset is primed for a slight alteration as your buddy announces the next round of shots are on him.

Oh, and what's this here? The bar has free pretzels? What a steal! Allow me to help polish off that pub mix for you. Cheers to empty glasses and empty calories! I don't care how many other grubby hands have been in this same bowl today.

There's more than a gratuitous amount of bacteria to worry about in those handfuls of Snyder's, however. Salty foods are provided to you *gratis* for one simple reason: to get you to buy more drinks. Sodium intake leads to dehydration, causing you to feel thirsty. And what's better to whet your whistle than an ice-cold brew? I feel like I'm narrating an episode of *Bar Rescue* right now. This same business sense applies to all of the paid fare on the menu as well. Bar food is salty, spicy, and infused with whatever it takes to have you clamoring quickly for cold refreshment.

You see, the profit margins for alcohol are far greater than that of food for the bar. Once upon a time in America, you could even find a full meal at the local pub for free. There may have been only one entrée to choose from on any given day, but nonetheless, your midday meal came with no sticker price. You may have heard the phrase "there ain't no such thing as a free lunch." Well, this is where they had you. While the edibles came at no cost to you, the one drink minimum attached to the deal was. If you had two whiskeys before returning to work for the afternoon, the saloon made out just fine. *Come again tomorrow, we have tuna salad on rye!*

This simple, but very effective manipulation of your consciousness applies not just to the local watering hole, but nearly every venue where an adult might come into contact with alcohol. Have you ever been to a baseball game? How about a trip to the cinema for that newly released film? Peanuts, popcorn, and nachos all plead your taste buds to fork over an additional $7 for your soft drink of choice. Even your favorite airline will hand out bags of free peanuts if you'll continue swiping your card for shot after shot of Johnny Walker. Here's another little fun fact: the airline peanuts are even saltier than the ones you'll find on terra firm, because your taste buds are less reactive at higher altitudes. It may not only be the flight jitters that keep you pressing the call attendant button.

- **Infomercials**

Back to the subject of television, no doubt you've seen the commercials promoting easy weight loss by just eating the food they send you in the mail. I'm looking at you, Nutrisystem. *Just eat, and eat! It's that simple!* Celebrities are adamant to share with you their personal secret to shedding those pesky pounds. I'd say they're motivated by the million dollar endorsements being thrown at them. *Chocolate cake? Pizza? Cheeseburgers? I don't have to stop eating any of the things I love!*

First of all, I can't imagine the preservatives necessary to keep that food fresh for the weeklong trip across the country. Assuming you actually receive what you ordered when the mailman drops off the box, you still have to get past the taste of all that "healthy" comfort food you asked for. If your meals are even marginally more palatable than the box they shipped in, there's a good chance you'll be itching to supplement your daily allotment with some good old-fashioned home cooking. *Just eat, and eat!*

One of the more difficult psychological hurdles to overcome is passing on food that promotes itself as healthy, where the opposite may be true. Honey Nut Cheerios has long advocated its heart-healthy product, promising to reduce the cholesterol of people who eat their tasty o's. A big heart is stamped right on every box, measuring nearly as big as the honeybee himself. General Mills reminds you that their cereal is not a standalone product, but part of a balanced breakfast. Okay, so I'll throw in two eggs over easy, four slices of bacon, and a pile of hash browns to make it "well-balanced". Somehow, by 8:30 in the morning, my heart is not exactly beating with pumps of joy. Beware of the health boosting labels. Just because your corn flakes have the daily recommended amount of fiber in each serving doesn't mean that it won't kill you in other sinister ways.

Don't get suckered in by the late night infomercials either. These 30-minute spots are masterfully crafted to make you hate life and shell out *ONLY $19.95* for a gimmicky contraption that sits on shelves and under beds in homes countrywide. *Six-Minute Abs! The Perfect Pushup! And who could forget the Shake Weight!* It's a common rationale to expect returns on an item just because you invested hard-earned money into it. Dialing the phone, you think, "I'm going to get every last penny out of this Ab Roller!" Then, when the UPS man shows up at your door, you're hesitant to even go search for the box cutter. Think I'm wrong? Find someone who actually learned a new language after spending $500 on

Rosetta Stone software.

If you're like me, then you don't even want to pretend like you're going to exercise. Even if I do have a new toy in the house, it's still more exercise than slunking from the couch to the fridge. Why can't I just take a pill to lose weight? *Hydroxycut, SlimQuick, Lipozene; one capsule every day and it's off to the buffet!* If you buy into that line, I got a hell of a deal on a bridge upstate. These supplements are little more than glorified energy bumps that "may" augment your daily activity levels. It can add a little pep in your step every morning, but what you do with that little spark of energy is what really matters.

Recently, I saw a product advertised by the name of Sensa. It's a powder that comes in a saltshaker, and all you have to do for it to work is sprinkle a little slim salt on whatever you eat. By the miracle of modern science, this magic dust purportedly reduces your appetite and makes it difficult to eat a massive meal. If a normal dining experience entails devouring an entire DiGiorno pizza in one sitting, now you're going to be content after inhaling only three quarters. Rather than encourage a shift towards leaner foods, Sensa prides itself on the fact that you can eat whatever your heart desires. The ineffectiveness of the magic salt becomes clear quite rapidly, and before long you're wondering why you're salting your Dairy Queen Blizzards. *And… what do you know! Not long ago, the company behind Sensa was fined by the FTC for false claims about weight loss. Who could have seen that coming?*

But check out the results on some of those featured testimonials! The before and after photos speak for themselves. *This product must really change lives!* The truth is, what you see is most often a play on photography. Aside from any Photoshop enhancements, what the producers don't clue you in on is the fact that the subjects chosen for a particular infomercial are already ripped specimens. Those "before" pictures you see are actually taken after the "after" pictures. Yes, the fat and bloated former selves of the past they show you are photos taken *after* the initial shoot. The inventors of new fitness equipment simply don't have the resources to track real-time results on a clinical level. It doesn't fit into either their budgets or their deadlines. You may notice in the fine print of their commercials that they explicitly state, "results are not typical" or "results may vary." If these little snippets of text were to be absent on screen, customers far and wide would sue these gadget manufacturers right out of the industry (and they still have). We, as consumers, expect products to deliver the outcomes depicted on our screens, regardless of whether or not we put any of our own work into it.

Jenny Craig and Weight Watchers pioneered the trend that other firms like Nutrisystem relishes in today, pushing clients to buy meals sporting their labels on the box. If you happen to be shy, Weight Watchers has an additional, infinitely more embarrassing program for your self-conscious form. *How about a humiliating public weigh-in every week?* Throw in a little public shaming in a room full of self-righteous strangers, and you're sure to drop those pounds like a sack of bricks! Besides, everything is so easy when all the food and drinks have a "points" system. *According to this chart, coffee has no points? Be right back, I'm going for out for a Venti Caramel Frap.*

- **Fat Acceptance**

Rather than subjugate your soul to the mercy of a corporate weight loss enterprise, why not support a non-profit organization that stands on a platform against fat discrimination and for the assimilation of overweight people into greater society? Yes, I recently learned that this is, in fact, a thing. The National Association to Advance Fat Acceptance (or NAAFA for short) is a group that focuses its resources on romanticizing the image of fat citizens everywhere. NAAFA believes that the multi-billion dollar dieting industry has perpetuated society's discrimination against fat people, and further believes in the self-empowerment and pride of their unique nutritional choices.

While it is certainly cruel to harass other human beings and their outward appearance, I can't help but think an organization like this is run by people living in the seventh hell of denial. Tomorrow, I should go out and register my own non-profit, the American Association to Advance Alcoholic Acceptance. *Five A's are clearly better than three; your argument is invalid. If I choose to play Edward forty-hands on a nightly basis, I am merely expressing my personality. You should treat me like the respectable alcoholic that I am, because I say so. Come join us Monday mornings at 11:00. We hand out bottle cap medallions at our weekly meetings for the everlasting binger.*

The people subscribed to these mentally ill movements have role models too. NAAFA's primary idol of worship? None other than the classic beauty, Marilyn Monroe. Why is that, you might ask? Ms. Monroe was the bombshell blonde of her time, a woman who millions of young ladies aspired to be like. Well, the people of NAAFA and similar others become giddy with joy when they get to point out the fact that at one time in her life, Marilyn was a size 16 with a near 40" waist. Many professionals would consider that quite overweight, or even obese. And that's where the cultists of today cite their devotion. Marilyn was the ultimate sex symbol, and a fat one at that. Therefore, if Marilyn was obese and an object of lust, why can't I be?

Unfortunately for these fat pseudo-historians, two inaccuracies are at play here. For one, Marilyn Monroe was not obese by any stretch of the imagination. She may have added on a couple of pounds at one point or another, but so do many celebs. The truth is, Ms. Monroe's beauty can be attributed to her unique bodily structure. She had a remarkably accentuated hourglass figure, so much so that tailors had to go to extra lengths just to fit her abnormal shape. She was indeed a rare beauty, but not for the reasons that fat acceptors believe. Monroe had real curves, unlike what the manatees of today are flaunting.

- **Fashion**

The other key point, one that continues to fool people worldwide, is the chronologic variations in clothing size. A size 16 in the 1950's isn't the same size 16 women will find at a

Forever 21 today. In present times, that size is much larger, which is yet another intentional act in marketing. In America especially, the size of clothing has been relabeled over the years to accommodate a proportionately growing populace. Companies have figured out that people will shop other brands if they don't fit in the same clothes at age 36 that they did in college. "I'm a size 12, goddammit. Aeropostale is wrong! Oh look, these Lane Bryant skirts fit just right." Denial is assuredly one of humanity's strongest traits, and savvy clothiers have capitalized on that fact. It's a race to the bottom, and some companies that haven't readjusted their sizing run the risk of losing customers to more accommodating brands.

Your clothing choices can be a direct reflection of your internal state of mind. If you're bopping around in a loose fitting t-shirt and gym shorts all day, how motivated can you be to live the life of a successful human being? Your casual attire may be appropriate for lounging around the house all day. Anything classier than a Wal-Mart, however, requires that you at least take some form of pride in your dress standards. You can't feel like a million bucks without dressing the part. When the business card of your multi-billion dollar firm reads "I'm CEO, Bitch," feel free to wear Spongebob pajamas to the meeting of the partners.

Many fashion brands are discouraged from weaving apparel that fits bodies of irregular shapes and sizes. The very image of a clothing company is often tailored around athletic or sporty individuals. Finding Nike or Adidas clothing in anything larger than a 2XL size can be a downright chore. Perusing through the local mall, you'll be hard pressed to find many stores that accommodate your larger frame. Sure, they have outlets like Casual Male XL and Lane Bryant, specifically geared towards oversized figures. These stores don't carry a wide variety of items that necessarily fit your sense of style, though. Premium companies participate in a form of selective discrimination by shuffling you away from marquee stores in favor of attracting trimmer clientele. This discouragement means you'll have fewer clothing options and the feeling that you can't really dress the way you would prefer.

Hip brands engage in other practices that purposefully forbid obese customers from donning their apparel. Brochures and advertisements, especially those of Abercrombie & Fitch, Hollister, American Eagle, and other similar tailors, feature young and trendy models. The projected image is that "you're fat, therefore you have no business wearing our clothing." The smug, subtle message perforating these advertisements is critical to competitiveness in certain niches of the market. If teenagers and college kids aren't sporting their brand's affiliation, companies risk falling back on brand-unaware seniors or facing altogether obscurity. Clothiers would rather (and often do) burn their unsold stock than see their clothes donned by society's undesirables.

The easiest way to scare off old and fat fashionistas is to manipulate the sizing of the clothing itself. Many customers, especially those who are body-conscious, would rather wear a size 2 from Torrid than a size 8 from Banana Republic. Though these items of clothing may be the exact same size in measurement, the end user perspective from wearing a shirt with a larger number on the tag is one of shame. Winning at clothes shopping is like winning at golf; the lower the score the better. If I go to Fatburger for lunch and only order a medium burger, I feel like I'm restraining myself. Though a Big Mac from McDonald's is roughly the same size, as long as I'm not going all out on the 2lb. XXL from Fatburger, I feel like a successful dieter.

Heavyweights are shunned simply for choosing to wear specific types of clothing that wouldn't get a second look otherwise. *Who wears short shorts?* Not I, but plenty of men and women out there do. It's common to find athletic types showing off a little extra skin, but that doesn't deter a certain subset of the porpoise population from letting it all hang out.

Midriffs, sundresses, tank tops, spaghetti straps, and short skirts are items privy to those who don't skip leg day at the gym (or any day, for that matter). If you went to Cheesecake Factory last night, it is lawfully prohibitive for you to wear anything but sweatpants or dark jeans for the next 10 days. Nobody wants to see your cottage cheese thighs pounding the pavement, sending Jurassic Park T-Rex shockwaves through my drink as you walk by.

    A select few deputies in the fashion police department have valid points. The goal of fashion is to accentuate the highlights of your unique figure and cover that which may be unflattering. Fat people can be stylish, in fact even more so than a good portion of Skinny Minnie's. Adele is a great example. No one argues the fact that she isn't of ideal weight, but she is definitely beautiful in her own right. When she dons a form-appropriate dress or gown, Adele gives off the aura of a stunning woman as she belts out her classic hits. If she decided one day to show up in a compression tank top and yoga pants, there's no doubt that she would be deafeningly rebuked clear out of the Royal Albert Hall.

    There's much to gain from taking pride in one's appearance. This is America, and I know that gives you and me the right to wear whatever the hell we want, whenever and wherever the hell we want. There are consequences to these actions, however, just as with other choices in life. If you insist on wearing as little clothing as possible, wouldn't you rather do it while eliciting looks of jealously, rather than scorn?

    I can't even begin to put into words the feeling I had when I put on the first pair of jeans that had a waist size less than the length of the inseam. From an all-time high of 48", reading that 33" x 34" tag on my new pair of Levi's was something I could only have dreamed of only a few short years ago. My grandmother died in December 2012, after a long struggle with her ever-deteriorating health. I very much wanted to attend her funeral, as she was very dear to me. The only problem was, none of the suits I had in my closet even came close to fitting. I scurried across town looking for an adequate replacement, and I found myself encountering an altogether new fashion problem. I was *too* tall and *not* fat enough. Joseph A. Bank only had the equivalent of a midriff in their armoire. The local big and tall outlet only had clothes for big *and* tall people, not big *or* tall. It took a visit to five different stores, but I finally landed a good two-piece at Burlington's, of all places. It turns out fat people aren't the only ones discriminated against when it comes to shopping.

No doubt you've passed the dozens of periodicals in the supermarket that pride themselves on living healthy lifestyles. *Fitness, Shape*, and other health-oriented magazines grace the checkout lines of grocery stores everywhere. That cart you pulled to the front is already full of Cheetos and Oreos, so you might as well take some advice on how to work that off later. The models featured on the covers would have you believe that they never enjoyed a cheeseburger in their lives. Their perfectly toned, tanned figures are laughing at you through the page, screaming at you to buy into whatever tips or tricks they have to offer you on page 36.

It's a devilish trick, employed by countless publishers, but it works. Magazines snare you into thinking that you'll be able to transform your body into the idolized human specimen just by reading and applying the "Top 10" techniques in one article. The truth is, just about every picture plastered across those full page spreads are doctored in some way. Photoshop allows even the most grotesque among us to shine in the photo booth. Every zit, pimple, pockmark, scar, varicose vein, stretch mark, dimple, and pore can be erased with the wave and click of a mouse. Airbrushing allows a body's natural curves to be accentuated in anatomically impossible ways. The camera may be feared for its ability to add 10 pounds, but a creative designer with an iMac has the power to shed 25. This unattainable perfection, held in our society to be the embodiment of normal, is attributable to feelings of shortcoming and self-consciousness for the majority of us who do not fit anywhere near the envisioned modicum.

- **Big Box Stores**

It may come as a surprise for some that the supermarket wasn't always an integral part of our communities. For a very long time in human history, men and women had to venture into nature to acquire sustenance. Men hunted wild game, not just for sport, but also for essential protein to supplement the diets of their towns and villages. Men and women both worked hard on plots of land to scour for essential vegetables and fruits. For city dwellers, acquiring these foods meant venturing to the local bazaar. You may have to go everyday, because there was no refrigeration to keep food fresh, and certainly no Chevy Suburban to haul a load of family groceries with.

In today's world, the local conglomerate grocery store is stationed on every corner. Preservatives and refrigeration advancements allow us to stock up enough food to last for months at a time. Stores will even deliver food straight to your fridge (for a fee, of course), rendering the acquisition of food nearly an obsolete task. Walmart (and even Amazon) are working on the logistics of delivering fresh groceries to your door at the whim of a click. Soon, autonomous drones could be delivering your Ding-Dongs. Convenience is a niche in which all companies aim to position themselves. The less effort it takes for you to purchase, the better.

More popular now than ever before is the sedentary lifestyle, the art of doing nothing. The less effort required doing anything and everything, the better. No longer chastised as laziness, it's an innovation in the name of efficiency and timesaving. It wouldn't surprise me at all if some Americans voluntarily use bedpans just to save the march to the porcelain throne. You don't even need to head out to Walmart for half of the things you need anymore. Amazon.com has got your back, bringing an ever-increasing number of household items straight to your front porch. Oftentimes, they do it for even less money than your local big box store, and you pay little to no shipping costs to boot. Sure, this is a dream come true for many, but think of all the exercise you're missing out on while walking around the store for an hour. It could be the most activity your body gets all day.

As an aside, the mere act of sitting in a chair has become its own health epidemic of late. It is estimated now that the average person spends a full 9 hours a day on their haunches, more than the typical 7 hours spent sleeping. In general, that means individuals are in a position of rest for the majority of the day. These unprecedented inactivity levels, largely spurned by the advent of the Internet, correlate with a 40% increased likelihood to die in the next 15 years. Sitting causes fat-burning enzymes to shut down 90% of your metabolic processes, further tempering the chances of weight loss.

- **Membership Warehouse Clubs**

Everyone knows you can save money when buying your favorite foods in bulk quantities. Thankfully, wholesale clubs are plentiful in much of America to serve the needs of citizens with larger than average appetites. Store like Costco and Sam's Club don't understand the meaning of a single serving. Everything from spare ribs to socks can only be found in quantities that can indulge a family of 20 with ease. Value size is the name of the game, and club members can save hundreds, even thousands of dollars with wise purchases.

What initially seems like a great bargain over the competition of your local supermarket may end up a huge loss to your health. You may not particularly desire to eat a bucket's worth of nacho cheese over the course of the two weeks upon opening it. However, if you don't, the expired leftovers equate to a net loss on your budget. Eat your money's worth, or why bother driving the extra mile to the warehouse in the first place? Eating what you bought from Costco is not only a practice of indulgence; it can become a downright chore. No single person should ever need to grocery shop at one of these monolithic stores. In reality, the pounds you save by trashing your leftovers probably equates to greater monetary gain in the long run. This situation is a classic scenario of penny-wise, pound-foolish logic.

- **Girl Scout Cookies**

Solicitations for the famished dollar inundate us everywhere, even right at your doorstep. One of the more popular fundraising promotions in our nation is the distribution of Girl Scout cookies. Arriving but once a year, a scout going door-to-door pawning their sweets is a time-honored tradition. They entice you with their sweet smiles and the promise of helping out your community. The turd in the punchbowl is that you have to pack on a few extra pounds to help your neighbors. Don't think you can buy just one box either! The life span of a box of Samoas at my house is about 8 minutes flat. And it's not just the girls who want a slice of your charitable income. Police organizations, high school clubs, and other non-profit groups sling delectable treats to the masses on a regular basis.

- **Fat Camps**

Overweight children of slender adults undergo a special kind of pressure from his or her parents to conform to their standards. You may find yourself staring at a pile of brochures when you're coming home from school one fine spring afternoon. What are they for, you ask? Well, the infographics laid before you are all about getting you amped up for the upcoming summer vacation, one you will be spending at your choice of highly-acclaimed fat camps. That's right, you and 400 other disappointing offspring are in for the experience of a lifetime! Just look at all the smiling faces on the covers of these pamphlets! Who knew kids like me could have such a kick-ass time away from the Candy Crush and Xbox?

What looks to be a summer of fun is sure to detour rather quickly into a hellacious affair. Fat camp? The alumni would attest that it's more akin to boot camp. Just get one thing straight. You are there because somewhere along the line, you fucked up. No one living a picture perfect life has ever crossed within 50 miles of one of these dietary reeducation camps. The food *will* be healthy. The days *will* be long. You *will* bunk with 20 other sweaty sacks that breathe just as much out of their ass as they do their mouth. Fun and games? No, run in chains. Welcome to the suck. You've been at Camp Carb for three days and you're already homesick, and there's still over seven weeks left to go.

The concept of a retreat for people who share a common goal seems like a great idea, in theory. Everybody is there to lose weight, retrain their lifestyle approaches, and generally feel better about themselves. Judgment has no place in these camps, for you all share the same deficiency. You would be the pot calling the kettle black, so to speak. However, the counselors and administrative personnel who operate the establishment have no such limitations. They are free to ride your ass all day over that jelly donut the camp counselor found in your locker.

Your biggest enemy at weight loss camp is that of your

fellow camp attendees. In an ideal world, your collective mindset would evolve concurrently with your peers and dieting would become second nature. Unfortunately, the overweight children at fat camps are largely devoid of self-control, and breaking the habits that have been instilled already at such an early age is unattainable for many. As a result, kids are going to fight tooth and nail to continue indulging on the very treats they hope to rid themselves of. You would think having a support group with likely-afflicted members would serve to boost confidence in kicking a habit, when in reality you are hanging out with a whole new room full of drinking buddies. The best place in the world to find drugs may be the person sitting next to you in Narcotics Anonymous. As for the place to find Snickers and Butterfingers when you're in the forest, six hours away from home? Right under your bunkmate's bed would be a great start. Expect to pay triple to your friend what you would at the Circle K, because these sugary snacks are explicitly prohibited at camp. Black market sweets could amount to a full time job for savvy young entrepreneurs, profiting on the backs of their compatriot's health and happiness.

- **The Gym**

Speaking of getting the kids in shape, what was *your* New Year's Resolution? For most of us, the answer to that rather open-ended question is to exercise more. Gyms are packed after the holidays, full of hard chargers who have *had it up to here* with their appearance. Fitness centers embrace your newfound resolve with open arms. It's the fitness Black Friday. *Come to our gym, your membership is waiting for you! It's open 24 hours a day, so now there's no excuse for not having enough time.* These clubs hawk annual memberships at reduced rates, because hey, if you're really committed then you're going to be showing up past mid-January, right? Planet Fitness even lets you sign up online, what a convenience! Good luck finding an open machine during the first week of the New Year. You're going to be encountering a ton of likeminded individuals clamoring for that same weight bench.

The gym is selling you nothing more than a fat tax, a monthly-billed sting to your self-confidence. If you really want to get in shape, you're going to want to bring a friend. Better yet, find out where your athletic buddies go to keep in shape and go with them sometime. If you're not ready for it, the gym can be a pretty intimidating place. It's not exactly a beginner's best place to start. There are rats that have been maxing out the equipment ever since they learned to use a syringe, and it's more or less their home away from home.

You don't belong. The gym is where fit people stay fit. If you're not ashamed of getting some dirty looks as you struggle with the lightweights, then go for it. If you're like me, and don't enjoy showing your gut in front of the pretty ladies on the elliptical, then you may want to stave off the pro circuit for now. Work your way up to it and you'll be far more likely to remain a dedicated member, instead of a fee-contributing silent partner.

- **Equipment Failures**

Feeling unwelcome at the gym is one thing, but to be ostracized from certain activities at home and around town is just that much worse. Many items you find at the house can be downright fatal or cause serious bodily harm. Ladders, trampolines, diving boards, and many other seemingly innocuous products can buckle under stress without warning. Plastic lawn chairs are something I especially loathe. Those cheap ones can't support much more than 150 lbs. before they bend and snap, causing damage to both my ego and my wallet.

The world around us was not designed to accommodate our larger statures. Airplane, stadium, classroom, theatre, and restaurant seating rarely fits the bill, or the butt. When these products are bought by businesses and venues, the optimal balance between price and function must be met. Unfortunately, the majority of people in most countries are still considered to be within a normal weight range, therefore products are geared towards satisfying their needs. Extra-strength items are less common and sell for a premium in small markets.

If you're overweight, it's simple. Lose the pounds, and you're in. If you're especially tall, however, well then you're shit out of luck. Watch your head, a mild concussion is waiting for you right under the next doorway. You must be *this* tall to ride the roller coaster, but not *that* tall to volunteer for your own beheading. How about a compact car for you, sir? *As long as it has a sunroof, count me in.* Light fixtures, fans, and other obstacles are pining to leave a shiner on your forehead. Then there's the forever-dreaded shower head. *Damn you shower head! I haven't washed my hair properly in a decade because of your dastardliness, shower head company. What is this, bathing for ants?* Tall people everywhere hate your cruel dwarf engineers.

- **TV Doctors**

Did I mention you should consult your doctor before setting out on your weight loss journey? By that, I mean *your* personal doctor, the one you see *in person*. Don't get pulled into the fad diets pushed by the medical experts you see on daytime television. More often than not, the bottom line today is exactly opposite to the doctrine you'll hear next week. *Don't ever eat carbs! Avoid fat at all costs! Wheat? No deal, go gluten-free now!* It's a fear mongering information overload, and it generally leaves us more confused than before we started watching.

Let's get one thing straight: there is no diet program that all doctors can agree upon. All bodies are different, and individual dietary needs are as unique as you are. I like to put weight loss doctors in the same category as psychiatrists. They hurl all sorts of ideas, suggestions, and prescriptions towards you at a blistering pace, and they bet on something sticking eventually. There is no silver bullet, in other words. The fact remains, despite all the advice and guidance these medical professions bestow upon you, a majority of patients still revert to their old ways following treatment.

It's a disinformation campaign, sparked by hot trends and breaking news stories. This spells ratings for syndicated cable health shows. An independent research lab from somewhere you've never heard of releases their ambiguous findings on the health effects of one variable versus a control group. Newsflash: drinking a gallon of Coca-Cola every day for a year correlates to excessive weight gain! *Who would've thunk it? I can never have a soda again!* Next week comes around. *Oh my god, wheat is poisonous! I guess the Cake Boss is just a mass murderer, offing Americans one wedding reception at a time.*

The quintessential teachings of the great Dr. Phil take the practice of asinine preaching to a whole new level. "It's time to get real about fat, or get real fat." Gotcha, Dr. McGout. Time to get real about denial is more like it. It's a good way to sell a book; I can't knock on that. In fact, I'm sure I could learn a thing or two to that end. If you ever get a chance to read this, Dr. Phil, I'd be thrilled to be on your show and comment on *real* weight loss. I have wares of my own to plug on TV.

You've probably also seen the insanely popular program, Dr. Oz. Broadcasting a full five nights a week, Dr. Oz dedicates his show almost exclusively to weight loss advice. Rife with metaphorical models, magic tricks, and weight loss experts, Dr. Oz covers nearly every angle of bodily function in hopes of educating his viewers about healthy habits and the consequences of not adhering to them. While seemingly altruistic in his intent, viewers will nevertheless process this information through their own selective listening filters.

Decoding an endless plethora of nutritional wisdom is simply not a communication skill most people possess. If all the audience takes from these shows is that they should eat more healthy fats and whole grains, what's stopping him or her from whipping up a tray of avocado lasagna every night? Though the fine gentlemen of television medicine possess medical licenses, take everything you ingest from these shows with a heaping spoonful of salt substitute.

- **Video Games**

I'll be the first to admit that I've played far too many video games in my lifetime. I remember getting my first Super Nintendo for Christmas, sparking a love affair with gaming that reels me back in to this day. Video games are an overweight person's best friend. It allows you to succeed in a world that doesn't judge or knock you for your appearance. For a span, you become the player you're portraying on screen, killing and maiming everything standing in your way.

Earning medals, rewards, and achievements for your successes, video games offer similar bounties to what you might expect when working hard at something in the real world.

Video games are an escape, a journey into a parallel universe that doesn't have the pitfalls or repercussions of taking any tangible risk. Shot in the head? Don't fret, you'll respawn shortly at the nearest checkpoint. Fell into a pit of fire? Buck up, Mario, Princess Peach is still waiting for you in the castle. While there is no penalty for losing, there is also no prize for winning. Other than showing off your mad skills to the long-distance friends you have on Xbox Live, your digital accomplishments mean little. They mean even less when the sequel to the game comes out next year.

You may have watched some of the sponsored gaming tournaments that offer cash rewards to winning players of some of the more competitive multiplayer titles. Starcraft, League of Legends, and Counter Strike have a huge professional gaming following today, and several elite players *do* clear serious loads of cash. This, however, is a full-time job for them. In fact, the hours invested into the gaming scene far outweighs any measurable salary they manage to scrounge from it. It is a dawn-to-dusk-to-dawn sort of occupation, and many spend 16 to 18 hours a day honing their skills to be ultimate tacticians. So dedicated to their craft, several of these real-time strategy perfectionists could theoretically orchestrate soldiers on a battlefield better than many officers in charge of real troops at this very moment.

Now, to showcase my personal relationship with video games, I will share this little tidbit with you. Not too long ago, I was one of the highest-level Call of Duty players in the world. When Modern Warfare 3 came out in November of 2011, I put life on hold and invested months of time in climbing the leader boards. I was ranked 32 out of millions in Free-for-All, arguably the toughest ladder in the game to scale. For me, it was a full time enterprise. I would wake up, shoot imaginary bad guys for 8 to 10 hours, rinse and repeat. I continued that cycle every day through mid-2012. I thought at the time that what I was doing was glorious, something that most men in my age range could respect. After all, Call of Duty graces just about every coffee table in the living room of males under 35.

In reality, if I had worked that hard at anything else, I could've turned all that time into real world cash. Hell, this book you're reading might have been on the shelves months ago. The opportunity cost spent chasing a goal that has no lasting value far underscores the worth of striving towards something that one day I could proudly hang up on my wall. I still like to play Call of Duty, though I've cut back considerably on the daily time invested. Okay, I got to #18 on the Ghosts leaderboard for a spell. But I'm slowly backing down again, I swear.

World of Warcraft was another addiction I found myself drowned in, particularly during the later days of high school. Looking back, the whole premise of the game is akin to a runway fashion show. It's all about showing off your epic gear in the major hub cities to people walking around the square. You can craft some of the best gear on your own if you learn a skilled trade. However, for the truly great stuff, you have to go raiding.

For those unfamiliar, raiding is an organized dungeon quest, carried out in groups of 10 to 25 players vying for the same great gear for their character. It's tough to maintain order in the ranks, so you usually only raid with the trusted members of your guild. Microphones are required, and attendance is mandatory every night. You can expect to invest at least 20 hours per week in raiding alone, and the bosses you slay don't always drop the gear that you really want. It takes real-world skills to be able to organize a successful guild.

Leadership, recruitment, human relations, and unyielding persistence are but a few traits shared by upper echelon officers. Again, if applied to any corporate setting, these bodies atrophying in front of a screen have the potential to be business powerhouses outside of the basement.

  The proliferation of the Internet has not only made games more engaging with live multiplayer; the Internet has caused the sheer number of games in existence to skyrocket. There are an infinite amount of games to try out these days, many free of cost. Before the turn of the century, there was a far more limited scope of released titles. Take it or leave it, these games were all you got. Segas, Nintendos, and Playstations had a set library of company-licensed titles to choose from, and the only multiplayer you could enjoy had to be with actual friends at your home. Unlike today, video game coding used to be an industry that only professionals with financial backing could compete in. Now, anyone can make a program on a computer with just a basic understanding of game mechanics, no coding required.

  The gaming industry, most recently, bas been taking off on smartphones and tablet computers. Mobile devices allow us to play our favorite games anytime, anywhere. I find a quick game of Family Feud on the iPhone fits timely with a morning bowel movement. Call me old-fashioned, but I used to find comfort in the fact that I could finish a game and be done with it, like a book on my shelf that I flipped through cover-to-cover. I've seen the scope of what this developer has to offer, and now I can move on to conquering the rest of the games. Flash-forward to today: *oh, you beat a game? Good for you, add on a hundred more levels for the low price of $4.99.*

Games of the past used to be a final product; bugs had to be fixed in beta or live on forever in an unpolished state. No longer the case, updates are rolled out as frequently as every day now. Developers can hastily push out crap to make their launch windows, and then clean it up later if they feel up to it. Beat a game recently that you just hate to put down? No worries, chances are that new maps, levels, and additions will be released sometime in the near future in downloadable content (DLC). These games just don't end. They are living and augmentable platforms that pluck our time and money from us an hour and a dollar at a time.

Remember when you used to have to go to Wal-Mart or Toys R' Us to buy video games? *Pepperidge Farm remembers!* (Wow, that's an old meme). For especially popular games, you might even have to journey all across town to find a copy of the title you want. Time and energy went into in thrill of tracking down hit games, a pastime long since forgotten. Today, games are a click away on your PC or home console. If you didn't preorder the game on Amazon or Gamestop months in advance, no worries. At 12:01AM PST on launch Tuesday, simply download the game straight to your hard drive. You don't even have to leave the couch to put the disc in. Now that's convenience at its finest.

    I remember the first time I ever played a game online. Age of Empires 2 was a very popular game when I was growing up, a real-time strategy experience that was furiously addicting to say the least. For the first few weeks I had it, the only game mode I ever bothered with was the campaign. You could play through the story as several various historical warlords, including Joan of Arc, William the Conquerer, and Saladin. Conquest on the digital battlefield was very satisfying, albeit mostly controlled by computerized intelligence. When I got bored with laying siege to the empires of old, I happened upon a secondary game mode: multiplayer. At first, I expected this game mode to be reserved for those who have their computers networked together in the same room, or even take turns on the same machine. What I got instead was an introduction to the glorious lobby of online matchmaking. *You mean I get to play against real people, across the globe?* Yes sir, indeed. *You can even chat with them during the match? Let the shit talking commence!* It may have been a total lag-induced stupor I was in at the time, but playing against random people from around the world on a 56k modem was a mesmerizing progression nonetheless. Villagers, to arms!

Study after study has shown violent video games to have no correlation with real world criminal acts. *That means they must be healthy, right? Can't stop playing now, I have to hit 6th prestige this weekend!* If there's one addition to the TV that is a greater time sink than channel surfing, it is the video game console. Some titles virtually mandate that you sit square on your couch for hundreds of hours on end, no joke. Many gamers live their lives in an *Inception*-like dreamscape, one that's much easier to delve into than real life. The trade-off for training to be a highly valued asset in the digital landscape can oftentimes reciprocate into deleterious work ethic in the analog world.

Gaming culture is infatuated with promoting Mountain Dew, Cheetos, and Taco Bell as if they're a critical life force. Got a six-hour raid to attend this evening? Better stock that mini-fridge, because you're going to need all the Game Fuel you can reach from your padded armchair. There's no real world benefit to playing as virtual players in a dimension that doesn't exist, and gamers know this. That rewarding feeling of excelling at a televised illusion is offset by an equally depressing realization that when the console shuts down, all perceived progress goes with it.

You slither to bed exhausted, sweaty, and running low on snacks. You've gained four pounds today, made zero money, and are likely retiring to a cold mattress in a dark room. You're no better off today than you were yesterday, or the week before.

Video games can be incorporated into a healthy lifestyle. That much I'm sure of. There are certain genres of games you should try to avoid, however. Don't get absorbed into role-playing games such as World of Warcraft, Elder Scrolls, Final Fantasy, or the like. These games either never end or require weeks of time to complete. RPGs are very difficult to just pick up and put down, as you'll seemingly get nowhere in the course of a couple hours of play. Also, try to avoid getting caught up in the ranking structure of some of the more popular first-person shooters. Call of Duty, Halo, and other shoot-'em-ups require an extensive amount of time just to break into the next rank. There are thousands of other people who have already broken your record, gained the achievements you think are worthwhile, or are just generally better players. The competition is fierce among no-lifers.

Instead, you may find a quicker fix with games that are designed with limits in mind. Sports games, for instance, require relatively short periods of time from start to finish. Fighting games can be even better. You're not likely to spend any more than half an hour in any given match. This allows video games to serve their intended purpose as stress *relievers*, rather than life-stagnating stress *inducers*. These games often have rank structures or unlockable characters too, though. I guess my advice would be to switch the games you play often, and try not to get caught up in the rat race. That new gun or character you want to unlock is generally not going to help you in multiplayer matches, and that's because publishers are adamant about supporting game balancing, a cornerstone in providing a fair experience for all players, new and veteran.

Finally (and this one's important), don't place too much faith in video games that promise weight loss through motion-based controls (i.e. Kinect and Wii motion). Some of the titles like this that I know of are the Wii Fit, Just Dance, or EA Sports Active. These games sell you large controller pads or motion sensors that you have to plug into your console, and they often cost upwards of $100. However, you're tempted to pay whatever the price is, because how great would losing weight playing video games be? Talk about a win-win scenario. You turn it on and have a refreshing workout the first time playing it. What happens all to often, though, is that the first time playing a workout game ends up being the last. Let's get real: what is the replay value of a game that kicks your ass up and down the street by design? When I turn on the Xbox, I can either throw in a game that makes me exercise, or I can play Halo. *Decisions, decisions.* I wouldn't be at all surprised if GameStop has a graveyard piled full of old dance mats and Wii Fit boards that people have pawned back for pennies on the dollar.

- **The Internet**

The Internet has grown into an enormous assemblage of entertainment sources. Porn aside, one can spend an entire day surfing the web and never view a familiar page. News articles, memes, and YouTube consume many a persons' entire existence. The Internet can take you all over the world without ever leaving the comfort of the sofa. Remember taking a trip down to Blockbuster to rent the latest films? It certainly has been awhile for me. The likes of Hulu, Netflix, and Redbox have all but eaten up the video rental business. The store comes to you now. And, unlike physical locations, you're not going to leave disappointed when the shop runs out of it's five copies of the latest Transformers.

Finding a suitable time sink online isn't limited to movies and TV shows, either. Oh, no, there are endless branches of the World Wide Web that are just waiting to be uncovered. Facebook, Twitter, and a whole host of other social media platforms allow us to experience the lives of our friends and family, without actually sharing any time with them. Today, we can live vicariously through the exploits of others unlike ever before. *Oh, cool, you got married last weekend? Congratulations! Let me spend the next 45 minutes browsing the 212 photos you uploaded. I know you invited me to be there two months ago, but that day I just had far too many beheading videos I'd rather watch instead.*

If you have a particular hobby that you can't get enough of, you're likely to stumble upon forums populated with strangers who share that common passion. Do you love your car? Of course you do, it is a man's pride and joy just as much (or more) than any children of his. Want to learn how to change the power steering fluid without coughing up a paycheck to a thieving mechanic? Join the Camaro forum, the Jeep forum, or even the Ford Pinto forum. If you can't find what you're looking for in the search box, just ask away. Before you know it, help will pour in to assist your cause. The rabbit hole doesn't stop there, either. If you like working on cars, you probably love racing them. Why not take a look at the NHRA or F1 forums? How about a racing video games forum? Are gas prices out of control? Let's find out at GasBuddy where the cheapest gas in town is.

No matter what happens to be on your mind, the Internet is there to provide. Available 24 hours a day, whenever we need it, sometimes our infatuation for knowledge causes ill effects in our lives outside the interwebs. You'll try to go to sleep around 10 PM so you can have a full night's rest for the long day ahead. But wait a minute! You just stumbled upon a highly thought-provoking thread at 9:52 PM, extending 172 pages deep. Looks like you might be catching yourself staring at a sunrise before you ever catch a wink of shuteye.

The 24-hour news cycle ensures that we'll never have a dull moment again in world events. It takes enormous willpower to unglue our eyes from the screen during any kind of breaking news. I find myself altogether enthralled with mashing the refresh key for one more post, one more little snippet of information I haven't yet seen. When you hear about events like the Boston bombing, Christopher Dorner, or the weekly school shooting, it can be near impossible to tear your eyes away from the screen. What's important to remember is that, while tragic, most of these crises have no direct impact on your life. You're voluntarily sacrificing your time and emotions by fretting over one malady where countless unreported others exist. Sulking on the couch in shivers instead of going for a walk is not going to bring back the brain-dead woman on the ventilator. Is that a bit heartless? Perhaps, but I'm here to help you with the problems that you actually *have* control over.

4

The Pharmaceutical Industry

Of all the organizations promoting unhealthy lifestyles to the general public, the ones that should be rooting for you in the stands should be America's pharmaceutical firms, right? After all, their primary goal is to cure the ailments of the general populace. Well, answer me this little riddle then if you would. How might pharmaceutical companies be profitable if their products solved all of their customer's problems? If that scenario were to become reality, these corporations would soon cease to sell their products and close their doors for good.

No, the companies manufacturing pharmaceuticals are perhaps among the seediest in existence today. You see their commercials running on television all the time. Half of the 30-second slot is set aside just to run off the deluge of side effects people are experiencing after taking said medication. *"Got a headache?"* your doctor asks. *"Here you go, one of these pills and you won't be able to feel your head for a week. Oh, and by the way, don't worry about that eczema, sore throat, heartburn, and anal* seepage you'll be dealing with over the next couple of days. That's normal. Everybody gets that. While you're in my office here, I'm going to go ahead and prescribe you three other medicines just to handle those 'minor' inconveniences. You'll soon be right as rain. And if not, just come back next week. We'll try a different cocktail."

Before you know it, you'll have more medications in your vocabulary than the old widow at the bingo hall. That which started as a lesser health concern can quickly escalate into numerous instances of medicinal dependence, serious illness, or worse. The medications designed to treat your side effects each have their own additional side effects, and the prescription pad soon reads more like an algebraic equation than a game plan. When you leave your health in the hands of a doctor, just know that many primarily care for you because your visits bought him a summer home in Malibu. If you're suddenly cured and require no further assistance, how is he going to swing the mortgage payments?

America is the most heavily medicated country in the world. We have been conditioned to believe that the FDA has our best interests at heart and all medical deficiencies can be cured with a tablet or pill. The United States is one of only two countries to even permit medicines to be advertised on television (the other being New Zealand). Every commercial ends with this or a similar statement: "Ask your doctor about [insert medication]." While many reasonable people would expect their doctor to prescribe the best meds to them, regardless of brand, patients often *do* ask for that specific one. And doctors are more than willing to prescribe what you saw on TV, just to appease their customers. Even if what you saw is not the best chemical treatment for your particular ailment, the placebo effect may trick you into thinking that it is. After all, those paid actors on television look so happy and carefree. *Why can't that be me?*

The miracle of modern medicine is not in the ability to resolve illness, but how corporate interests have managed to hold your life in a metaphorical vice. The balancing act of keeping patients alive, but not cured, remains a critical element in the perpetuity of the industry. Their goal, above all else, is to make sure you keep making regular visits to your doctor. Every time your doctor rips a sheet off that prescription pad, either you or your insurance company is tearing out a fresh check to GlaxoSmithKline or AstraZeneca. Plugging our nation with fatty foods and creating medication that induces weight gain makes this feat an easy endeavor for American capitalists.

Obesity marches lockstep with a profusion of its own

related illnesses. Depression nears the top of that lengthy list. *No problem, we have many medications available for your choosing.* SSRIs constitute a great percentage of these so-called "happy pills", synthesized to make you impervious to sadness. Unfortunately, these medicines come with their own dish of side effects, weight gain chiefly among them. *Are we happy now?* Gone are the days of eating due to stress or anxiety. Now you indulge just because you are indifferent of the consequences. This is not to mention the added sexual dysfunction you may be experiencing. *I'm curious as to why you're still feeling dissatisfied with life. It must be time to switch up those meds again.*

Depression drugs do work in many cases, I can't discard that fact. Chemical imbalances exist in many of us, and Prozac may indeed be a godsend. But for those of us who are depressed for reasons other than a minor case of the blues, no drugs exist that make us forget what is an everlasting reminder in the mirror. Fat is forever. You have to transform the environment you exist in to emerge from the spiraling cycle of depressive thought. Pills alone make few among us truly happy.

Therapists rarely cure anybody. Even when the root of the cause is discovered and patients have a "moment of enlightenment", they typically fall back into their cyclical, destructive patterns. The principal objective of most psychiatrists, therefore, is to keep their clients from jumping off a bridge. Anything beyond that is a success story. Some will rebound, sure, and live a more fruitful and prosperous life. Most who are perpetually depressed, however, will continue to live within the same vortex of despair. How helpful can it truly be to have an outlet where you can share your darkest, deepest thoughts with a stranger? I thought that's what the Internet was invented for.

Other than feeling down on themselves, overweight adults may soon feel the sting of something else: diabetic syringes. Obesity plays a key role in the development of type 2 diabetes, an illness manageable only by implementing positive lifestyle changes. Testing and injecting will become an unwelcome routine, but your life will depend on this regimental commitment. You should be thanking your pancreas every day for regulating your insulin, or soon you may have to take extreme measures to do so consciously. With diabetes, blood sugar levels can reach dangerously low levels, and your only lifeline at times may be that cheesecake you've been saving in the freezer.

Extra weight can take years off your life, make no

mistake. If diabetes isn't serious enough, add in the heightened risk of heart disease, high blood pressure, arrhythmia, and sudden cardiac arrest to your list of reasons to get fit. And wouldn't you know it, even if you choose to do nothing about your weight, there is a prescription medication you can take to address every single one of these little cardiovascular pests.

You may one day require hospitalization, and isn't that a medical provider's wet dream! Obesity can wreak havoc on your entire body, not to mention your healthcare premium. Heart conditions may warrant costly surgical operations that involve the implant of stents and pacemakers. If arterial plaque doesn't stop your heart, wait 'til you see the medical bill! Spinal injuries, nerve damage, kidney stones, knee damage, bunions, gout; the list goes on for conditions that obesity contributes to. Diagnosing these abnormalities requires the use of x-rays, CT scans, MRIs, biopsies, or any other specialized and highly expensive test you can think of. Doctors realize that once you are under inpatient care, charges associated with your hospital stay are at their discretion. For urgent situations, though, patients simply have no other option.

Every little object in your hospital room is guaranteed

to have a charge associated with it. You know those little paper cups they put your pills into? Those don't cost more a few cents each (to the clinic, that is). But no, the hospital is likely to charge several dollars per cup, per dosing period. This will be listed on your bill as something along the lines of "medical administration device." Markups on simple products such as latex gloves or pens often reaches upwards of several thousand percent. Hospitals get away with these price-gouging tactics simply because they assume that you don't know any better. Most people just want to pay the bill, forget about their horrendous medical layover, and move on with their lives. The names of all the line items on the bill are so vague or ambiguous that those who wish to contest their charges don't even know where to begin.

5

Government's Role

More Americans now than ever before rely on governmental assistance to survive. Thanks to a shaky economy, the Supplemental Nutritional Assistance Program (SNAP for short) provides food income for an unprecedented number of citizens. It's not luxurious by any means; many families have a very hard time stitching together a full three meals per day for their households. This means the pricier, healthier commodities (such as fruits and vegetables) are totally off the table (kitchen table, that is). It remains far more costly for the agricultural industry to preserve and deliver raw plant food than it is to ship processed cans and boxed items.

For those receiving assistance, it's all about maximizing the return on your food to dollar investment. Pastas, ramen, beans, rice, and Spam are chocked full of the calories people need to stay satiated until sundown. You can buy fresh fruits and vegetables with food stamps if you wish. But for every 20 apples you buy, one box of spaghetti will supplant an equal amount of energy to your poor, starving soul. It is not an economically wise decision to eat healthy when you're living on the government dime, so many will futilely succumb to a life of lipids.

You would think that feeding the poor is the principal mission of charitable foundations in this country, but that is not the case. The poor eat plentifully. Drive around any inner city or urban area and you will know exactly what I speak of. Obesity has passed starvation as the larger humanitarian crisis worldwide. By restricting access to a balanced diet, the poor have just enough to spend on bulking sustenance. The government is then tasked with the burden of providing health care for the indigent obese, negating any perceived taxpayer savings by putting less money on the SNAP cards.

I was shopping at Walmart recently, picking up a couple things for the house. It was a routine stop, more or less. If you know how long the checkout lines at Wally World get, you know that what you thought was a 5-minute trip quickly turns into the greater part of a half hour. *I still don't understand why they have 30 checkout counters when only four are operational at any given time.* Anyways, for the protracted length of time I found myself waiting in line, I happened to get stuck behind two "curvy" middle-aged ladies, with an overflowing cart to accompany them, no less. Filled to the brim with Funyuns,

Cheetos, Hot Pockets, Coca Cola, and Mountain Dew, it was easy to see why menopausal hormones played only an Ursa Minor role in the formation of these planetoids. After the cashier had totaled up their comestibles, out it comes from the older lady's purse. An Arizona "QUEST" card (the catchy title for food stamps here) slides through the register, and off the moons go back into orbit. Now call me crazy (or ignorant), but wouldn't grabbing the store brand equivalent of these products free up some cash for a few vegetables in the mix? I guess that bag of Ore-Ida brand fries will have to suffice.

    Sadly, when families are on government assistance, kids are the ones to go hungry first. Mommy and Daddy always get enough to eat, but the kids often get left to fend for scraps at home. The government knows this, so many children from low-income families are privy to free or reduced cost meals at the local schools. Mystery meat and chicken nuggets abound in these subsidized institutions, raising your kids on a diet loaded with ample quantities of sodium and fat. The same realities that apply to the poorest citizens of our country face the budget-strapped educational facilities as well. Vegetables are a premium item that schools don't want to waste on kids, so pizza has been reclassified as a vegetable to dispel the concerns of health-conscious parents. The youth of America get hooked on this corpulent cuisine from a very early age, so the craving for anything else is largely nonexistent as they transition to adulthood.

The temptations of junk food extend far beyond the lunch lines. Vending machines litter our public campuses, a highly profitable side venture for educational institutions. Their quick access is perfect for students trying to nab a snack between classes. Many of these impulse buys are made due to stress, but migrating from one desk to the next every hour is not exertion enough to warrant a *Butterfinger*. Failed a test? Made a clown of yourself in front of your crush? A bag of peanut butter M&Ms doesn't care about that. M&Ms can only love, not chide.

Teachers are running their own games to make some extra scratch too. Refrigerators full of soda and cases of snacks are being wheeled right into the classrooms, turning a learning environment into a mini mart. Nothing can stop your teacher from giving an hour long, droning lecture on the symbolism of Rennaisance poetry. An ice cold Mountain Dew might just keep you from falling asleep, though. At the very least, it will probably stop you from writing a negative review about their course on Ratemyprofessers.com.

First Lady Michelle Obama has been on a march to

reverse the trend of childhood obesity in schools on various fronts, including replacing sugary sodas in the vending machines with healthier fruit and sports drinks. This may be a welcome shift in variety for the student athlete, but for the majority this constitutes little change in total consumption. Fruit juices often contain just as much sugar as sodas, and Gatorade or Powerade is chocked full of calories designed to fuel a large burn of energy from playing sports. Students may be under the impression that if the new drinks are healthier, then there should be no problem in consuming two a day instead of one. Reducing meal portions to shave calories off those lunch trays has the opposite effect as well. Kids go hungrier and sooner, beg for after-school snacks, and the children end up having four or five unhealthy meals a day instead of a square three.

That's okay; why not let the kids load up on all that brain food? They'll run it all off in gym class anyways. Not anymore. Classes in physical education are vanishing every year, and it's all in the interest of holding to the district's bottom line. State and federal funding is not allocated based on how many sit-ups the students can do (only in the military). No, the monetary floodgates only open based on the number of kids who occupy their desks and bubble in the right circles on the standardized test. You can't manage that with a trombone in hand, either. Core curriculum is all that manages to evade the classroom chopping block. Everything else is fair game. The National Football League has taken notice to this alarming trend, introducing its *Play 60* campaign to help stem childhood obesity and encourage kids to stay active in school activities, despite the forces working against them.

In my school, kids had a choice of whether to join gym class or participate in one of the fine arts. Being the obese sack of shit that I was, this option was a no brainer. I could be in the band, the chorus, or enrolled in theatre. I chose band, every time. I played alto saxophone for seven years in school. And let me tell you, it was by no means an adequate substitute for physical education. Marching once or twice a year in the hometown parade isn't anywhere near training for the Ironman triathlon.

Remember the USDA Food Pyramid? I'm sure you've seen the poster hanging in at least one of your classrooms growing up. *Eat two to four servings of fruit per day, and make sure you save room for an entire six to eleven loaves of bread at the bottom.* This guide that has permeated our collective knowledge of what good health means is largely unfounded in science, and it doesn't represent an average American diet in the slightest. So you know what the government did? They issued a new pyramid, only this time all the food groups are distributed equally. Moderation trumps everything else. Eat whatever you want, but make sure you eat equal amounts of all the other things. Your grandma knew more than most people give her credit for (everything in moderation). Have you even heard of this new pyramid, though? Not many people are even aware of this fundamental change in federally suggested dietary guidelines. If nothing else, I would say what they did only injected more confusion into the mix.

The slop they shovel onto the food trays at schools in abominable, without a doubt, but even these meals pale in comparison to the inedible fare served up at our nation's correctional institutions. If the confines and squalor of Con College don't immediately foster a bad mood, then chow time most certainly will. Just as those who are locked up in penitentiaries are likely to reoffend after they're released, the eating habits of the incarcerated are likely to translate to the outside world as well. The inmates privileged enough to have money put on their commissary accounts still may only feast on vending machine grub, a far cry from any semblance of freshness or health. The correctional officers knew the last thing you wanted was a tossed salad anyways!

While many convicts wisely make the choice to spend

their time on the inside working out and maintaining a fit appearance, those who pig out on Doritos and honey buns do little more for themselves than occupy a cot with a warm body. Delivering fresh produce to penal institutions is a hassle and a logistical nightmare. Besides, fat and lazy inmates are viewed as a good thing from the CO's standpoint. Though they may be larger, unfit inmates are likely to be more complicit to the demands exercised upon them through authority. They're too slow to put up a contestable physical defense. Plus, inmates receiving treatment for obesity related illness, through government-subsidized healthcare, keep the wheels of Big Pharma turning.

If you're lucky enough to make it to a real college, your food choices at arm's length become somewhat more reasonable. The cafeterias of adult students are big improvements over the lunch lines and hairnets of old, though the increase in variety spawns a whole slew of additional deathtraps. Unlimited refills at the soda tap, pizzas on pizzas, and a personal sandwich maker turn an institutional grind into a slice of Jabba the Hut's heaven. Sure, there's a full salad bar and a whole array of fruits to match. But in a setting where I can have three bowls of frosted flakes, four Dr. Peppers, and a slice of red velvet cake at 3 in the afternoon, making room on the tray for a bowl of greens somehow doesn't fit in the budget of stomach space.

The federal government is not only a large purchaser and provider of food itself. The feds also regulate the sale and specifications of food sold in the private sector. The Food and Drug Administration mandates food producers to list the contents of their products on the labels of every container they sell. Ingredients and Nutrition Facts are universal and generally accurate in detailing the contents enclosed therein, though these figures are no less confusing now than when they were introduced. Seriously, who can pronounce half of the ingredients on some of these packages? If you have allergies, the ingredients list can be a godsend in preventing a nasty reaction, if you know what to look for. But the rest of the names on the list leave us in a state of bewilderment, and we end up loading the grocery cart full anyways in a state of ignorant bliss.

Even more befuddling is the nutritional content charted out on the labels. Calories? Calories from fat? Sugar, sodium, monounsaturated fat? What do these mean to me, and what should I avoid? I'll tell you now that *calories are king*, but we'll save the specifics for a later chapter. What is important to find out is where those calories come from. Not all fat is bad, and not all sugar and carbohydrates are bad. Some of the healthiest foods have a nutritional label that reads like a pecan pie at first glance.

Restaurants are off the hook when it comes to disclosing the ingredients and nutritional value of their entrées, at least here in America. Who knows what evil lies deep within the Alfredo sauce of your Chicken Carbonara? Restaurant dishes are a brew of insidious wares. To announce their secrets to the world would be to reveal their trademarked recipes. This is not to mention that aggregating the nutritional stats requires costly and tedious compiling, especially for a small business. It's also nearly impossible to quickly assess a dish on special for one particular day. Fortunately, some of the more progressive nations have made it mandatory to at least display the calorie counts of their meals on restaurant menus. McDonalds has pioneered the trend here in the United States, offering complementary statistics to buck criticisms of pushing junk food unknowingly onto less-than-bright customers.

McDonalds isn't concerned with our personal health, however. People have become so outraged at the products the company offers that some even believe it's morally unjust. Many overweight patrons blame McDonald's directly for impacting their health, as evidenced by the several lawsuits that have been filed over the past decade. Yes, people have sued McDonalds for making them fat. Somehow, someway, Ronald McDonald has been force-feeding them into obesity and malaise. A few have even won preliminary injunctions, only to be tossed out later when the McDonalds A-Team defense squad and common sense take action. Seriously people, what did you expect to happen? You can't sue a business for over serving your lard ass (unless it's alcohol, of course).

New studies about the effects of displaying the nutritional information on restaurant menus have come out already, and the verdict isn't surprising. The numbers don't make any friggin' difference to overweight diners! The figures only help the people that count calories, patrons who are already likely living a healthier lifestyle to begin with. Less than half the people who were surveyed even noticed the numbers, and the amount of times they ate at the restaurant hadn't declined at all. When you order the two for $4 Big Mac deal just because you want to save a buck, chances are calories are the least of your concerns. Calorie counts at Mickey D's are about as effective as the lung cancer warnings on a chain smoker's pack of Newports.

Do you enjoy going to the movies? How about a nice

day at the ballpark? Don't even think about bringing that granola bar into the venue. First of all, it's against policy. And if you're caught, you'll be asked to leave. If you haven't had a chance to grab a bite before walking through the gates, prepare yourself for the onslaught of fat-filled fare your event of choice has to offer. Super jumbo chili dogs, extra large popcorn, and seven dollar soft drinks round off the total gamut of grub. The prices are going to be steep, as will the needle on the scale. But you know what? No matter what the costs are, you're going to pay it. What other choice do you have? Try sitting through a four-hour game in the sun without once grabbing for an ice-cold beer on tap. It's not happening here in Arizona, I'll tell you that.

You don't even have to get out of your rigid and backbreaking stadium seat to grab a bite, either. Vendors have been lugging huge bins piled high with fiendish treats up and down the rows for decades, eager to grab the price of convenience right out of your hands. They even have movie theaters now that will bring you full blown dinners at the push of a button, saving you the excursion down to the lobby.

These closed market venues apply to airline travelers, too. If you've been through an airport recently, you know that healthy food simply doesn't quell the jitters of a traveling business pro. Cinnabons, pizzas, muffins, and bagels own the space between the security checkpoint and the gates. *Oh no, my flight has been delayed 7 hours due to bad weather? Let's see if an apple from the newsstand will hold me over.* Yeah, I didn't think so. In three minutes you'll be waiting over in the line of shame at Cinnabon, inducing yourself into a diabetic coma for the duration of the layover.

Airlines are always finding new ways to take advantage of their weight-challenged customers. Many carriers now require that you purchase two seats if you happen to board their planes with an above-average girth. This seems only fair to other passengers, who would otherwise be suffocated being sandwiched next to you. Some even charge based exclusively on weight alone, whether or not you carry your weight well. That extra 100 or 200 pounds can easily cause the plane to burn several more gallons of fuel during international flights, an expense that budget-cinched airlines are eager to pass along to the customer. If you're a frequent flyer, these charges could add up rather quickly.

Cruise ships are not much better. In fact, they're worse for the reason that you're confined for several days before you ever reach port. The all-you-can-eat crab legs at the end of the buffet are sure to grab your attention before you even get a peek at the fruit arrangement. An orange may cure your scurvy, but carrot cake eases the homesickness. I still can't figure out why anyone would want to take a cruise in the first place. $12 margaritas and a free case of norovirus are not things I would chronicle as a fun way to spend a week's time off.

As a traveler, you don't even have to venture by air or sea to fall prey to the influence of pound-packing eats. Take a road trip out of town and you're likely to find yourself miles away from the nearest health spa. Billboard after billboard line the highways, pleading for you to exit left in two miles for a juicy Whopper to fill the tank of a weary wanderer. In unfamiliar destinations, the only trustworthy options available are those familiar entities you've become accustomed to. The Carl's Jr. in your hometown serves up the same six-dollar burger as the one in Gallup, New Mexico. The bathrooms should at least have the same standard of cleanliness. Most don't have the time or the willpower to make a detour through the grocery store to scour the aisles for something bodily beneficial. Gas stations and Qwik-E Marts are the traveler's grocer.

National infrastructure has forever changed the way we get from point A to point B. Before the construction of the national interstate system in the mid 20th century, going anywhere fast presented a serious challenge. Though many roads did exist, most were either narrow two-lane stretches or gravel-paved at best. Roadside breakdowns were more common than they are today, and the nearest service station was often a 15-mile hike away. Going for a drive, the next town with a restaurant could easily be a few hours off.

America has since become an entirely car-centered culture. With the exception of residents in New York City, most can't cruise a block down the road without loading up our 7 passenger SUVs and cranking up the tunes. Every restaurant in town is no more than a quick jaunt away, and the doggie bags we bring home after a five-course meal are still fresh when they get put it in the fridge. Many restaurants now have either a drive-thru or to-go parking, making a walk to the front door purposeless. Minimal effort on the customer's part is required in today's food scavenging. You can have dinners and desserts from your favorite restaurant shipped across the country, even the world. Key Lime pies from Florida, French pastries, and chocolates from The Netherlands will arrive at your doorstep in no time flat. Just click or call.

Worldwide, the perspective of transportation is far

different and actually far more economical. Residents of international cities are far more likely to rely on the local means of mass transportation, hitching a ride on subways or city trams. Seas of bicycles occupy any given corner, permitting riders to easily wind through narrow city streets. Carpooling is far more common, and the accompanying riders may have to walk or bike their way to the designated rendezvous point. Sure, many people still drive their own individual automobiles. Superhighways, including the German Autobahn, do service the need for speed. For shorter distances, though, physical modes of transportation still have advantages.

The landscape of restaurants and food retailers has shifted immensely due to the innovations in roadway systems in the later 20th century. National fast food chains were unheard of until McDonalds started franchising its empire. Restaurants in the past had to rely on local sources for ingredients in their dishes to ensure a stable shelf life from farm to plate. In the past, ensuring consistency across multiple locations would require a close proximity to those ancillary locations. Nowadays, semi-trucks full of identical products reach every franchise nationwide. The chicken McNuggets you order in Bangor, Maine are the same ones you'll find in San Diego. Nearly devoid of nutritional value, many of these mass-marketed processed and refined foods now reach all corners of the globe.

6

National Consequences

Have you taken a look at your health insurance premiums lately? They're going up again. American's health care system is under immense pressure from several demographic subsets, most notably the elderly, the obese, and the terminally ill. Failure to manage your weight is causing fees to soar for us all. If people of normal size have any credible reason to poke jabs at your appearance, this is it. You may be reasonably "healthy" now, but insurance adjusters are betting on your fat ass taking a turn for the worse sometime in the future.

Weight also affects fuel consumption, and the added supply to compensate for your fat ass translates into higher gas prices. Taking a plane home to visit your family for the holidays? When one person carries the weight of two full-grown individuals, more trips and stops have to be made to shuttle everyone along. Trains, buses, and cars all need that sweet fossil fuel to make the world go around. The finite supply available means higher fares and prices at the pump for all of us.

Americans are "too fat to fight." This is the stern warning our military's top brass are trying to get through our gelatinous skulls. Obesity has surged to such a rate that one in four young adults are simply too physically unfit to enter service for our country. That's a full 9 million potential recruits, saved by the bell. Taco Bell that is. Combined with the number of fighting age adults with criminal records, drug addictions, or lacking in a high school diploma, the summation of ineligible men and women soars to 75%. If our country were to face a serious national catastrophe anytime soon, the US government would struggle in drafting enough Americans to defend our home soil.

Obesity is a real and growing vulnerability to our national security. Freedom is not (nor ever will be) free, in any sense of the word. Somebody has to go and fight for your right to drive-thru Dunkin' Donuts. If you're not losing weight for yourself, do it for God and Country. You think China or Russia doesn't have a sufficient pool of able-bodied killing machines to pick from? Think again. All of the sophisticated military technology we possess today couldn't begin to supplant any door-kicking ground invasion in these countries (if there ever is a call for it).

Thanks to our vast capabilities in world dominance, military conscription is a tool utilized only during times of great need in our country. This is not the case in many other nations of the world. Military service is often mandatory for young males, requiring a non-negotiable commitment of two years or more. These countries have standards that must be upheld to ensure armed readiness, and this includes regular physical training. Malevolent behaviors learned in childhood are scrapped in favor of strict military discipline, preparing servicemen and women for a future of more sustainable habits and personal responsibility. Those who fail to maintain a certain level of physical activity may be separated with a dishonorable discharge, a sentence nearly as detrimental to one's future as a felony conviction.

Obesity not only impacts our safety in a broader sense, but it directly affects people at home who are already in a vulnerable state. Expressing your right to abuse handicap spaces and motorized shopping carts has a toll on the seriously disabled persons who actually require them. A Hoveround is not a mere convenience to your couch-prone self. It's a connection to the outside world for many otherwise-bedridden people.

I witnessed an incident a few years ago at a place by the name of Johnny and Hangus, a local sandwich shop in Fair Lawn, NJ. I saw a woman push her no-less-than 600 lb. husband in for a bite to eat, watch him inhale the largest cheesesteak on the menu, then roll him right back to the car. I'm not sure if I had more sympathy for the wife of this man or for the suspension on their poor little car. If requiring a push to the counter isn't a signal that you need a change, then maybe realizing the color of your face is matching the car as you fidget your way into your red sedan is enough.

Though most obese citizens have no other reason than their own lack of self-control to blame for their physical condition, some people legitimately cannot lose a single pound. No matter what changes in their daily regimen they choose to implement, genetic makeup and a select range of diseases offer little hope of ever living thin. Hyperthyroidism, PCOS, and diabetes chiefly among them, patients diagnosed with these conditions have a near-impossible time shedding the pounds. For hypochondriacs who diagnose themselves as having these weight-related illnesses, shedding the excuses is their primary ailment. Contrary to what many would have you believe, only a small fraction of the obese are cursed with the impossibility of change. Despite their convenience, extra-wide bathrooms stalls and automatic doors were not designed with your rump round in mind. The truly afflicted are rightfully deserving of their medical assistance, and it's a shame that so many others con themselves into believing that they do too.

    The glutton bug is not just a problem indigenous to America these days. Though the good old U.S. of A. ranks number one in the percentage of obese citizens, other countries are making alarming strides. Thanks can be given to the McDonaldization of countries, seen to corporate executives as little more than "emerging markets." The rest of the world wants a taste of the Quarter Pounder with Cheese we Americans stand proudly by, and they're going to get it. The United States no longer offers fast food chains the expansion potential necessary to sustain large multi-billion dollar enterprises. There is already a fast food joint at every intersection in our country. Adding more would only decrease the share of their own profits from the next closest restaurant. The United States has reached market saturation, so most of the new restaurants that chains are putting up here are merely existing locations being rebuilt.

    Instead of keeping operations centralized in the homeland, new franchises are jumping across the pond and opening doors in nations that have never before seen a drive-thru window. There are billions of people in Asia and other developing continents who are now being exposed to the eating habits of westernized society. Hundreds of new fast food restaurants are opening every year, and they're everywhere but America. *KFC, coming to a Nepalese village near you!* People who have survived on the diets of a hunter/gatherer for thousands of years are replacing their love of fresh fish and rice with Filet-o-Fish and large fries. Obesity rates in these nations, once known for fit and lean citizens, are now steadily rising.

7

Fat Acceptance and the Embracement of Failure

When I was growing up, I was genuinely confused about why I was overweight. It was natural for me to eat every meal until I could eat no longer. *Isn't that what everyone does?* I remember feeling like a king for downing those 10 piece McNuggets and Super Size fries back in grade school. Looking back now, it wasn't hard to spot that I was an idiot. I subscribed to the train of logic that the more I ate, the more of a "real man" I was. The only thing all that food made me was a real fat man. The Internet has even coined a term for this bizarre and irrational arch of thinking, known to many as simply "fat logic."

Fat logic is more or less a trove of excuses that overweight folks fall back on when others call them out on their unhealthy eating habits. Much in the same way drug addicts rationalize their behaviors, no matter how extreme it may appear to others, fat people are staunch advocates of their personal decision to knock back a double Big Mac meal deal and order a McFlurry to go. I've never witnessed a family intervention for obesity, but the A&E network sure as hell should start. *My name is Marcus, and I'm a food addict.*

When I was morbidly obese (God, I love phrasing that in the past tense), I believed many of these unsound ideas that fat people are somehow superior for being able to consume more than their lean counterparts. *Bigger means stronger, right? Stronger is better than skinny and feeble!* What I came to learn over time, though, is that "bigger" just means bigger.

I already mentioned the NAAFA organization earlier, the group of people who are committed to fat acceptance in society. Further than mere acceptance, however, many followers of this cult engage in practices of reverse fat discrimination. Sympathizers of this cause are quick to judge the eating and exercise habits of people of all sizes, including those of clinically ideal weight.

You may have heard about the Health at Every Size (HAES) movement. HAES is the idea that people of all shapes and sizes can, in fact, be healthy human beings. Forget the bad knees and Type 2 diabetes. Any condition you may have, short of a terminal illness, is little more than a casualty of your genetic makeup. Many supporters of HAES cite historical differences in societal views towards voluptuous citizens.

"Overweight people were viewed as more sexually attractive than skinny people in the olden days!" Yes, this was indeed true in many cultures, especially among women. Women with wider hips were seen as better equipped to birth heirs to their husbands. The advances of modern neonatal medicine were unheard of, and any complications that arose could not be rectified with a simple C-section or other life-saving procedure. Today, of course, these advantages have since been greatly mitigated and no longer justify the Jessica Simpson diet.

A few extra pounds was seen as more than just a leg-up in the baby making process. Spare tires on both men and women were associated with status and wealth. In the land of famine, the man with meat was king. Starvation has spelled death for thousands of malnourished souls over the ages, but having that little bit of extra reserve handy ensured you would live through the harsh winter. Doctors would even recommended their patients maintain a slightly overweight figure in the event that he or she developed Wasting Syndrome as a complication of Tuberculosis or other debilitating illness.

Fat tolerance is not a struggle towards some vision of equality. Rather, the movement generally exists as an all-out offensive between the fat and the fit. This is Thin Privilege, or TiTP, is a blog on the popular Tumblr website that showcases numerous examples of fat discrimination and how overweight people are treated like second-class citizens. "Thin privilege" is having second helpings at the buffet without garnering seething looks from your friends. Thin privilege is fitting comfortably in a restaurant booth, or taking up only one airplane seat. Thin privilege is not having to go to the local zoo for an MRI because the machines at the hospital have a 500 lb. weight limit. New filth like this is added to the page every day, and the posters are serious as a heart attack.

"Fat privilege," as it were, is the de facto opposing faction, with some of their claims being equally as fervent as the TITP posters. *Fat privilege* is getting a handicap-parking sticker because your 450 lb. frame can't hoof it to the Wal-Mart scooters. *Fat privilege* is living on the government dime because your obesity qualifies as a "disability." Taking up a seat and a half on that flight you paid only one ticket for? *Fat privilege again, bitch.* The circle jerk emanating from both sides is an ongoing war of attrition, though a war of *nutrition* may be a more fitting struggle.

The deluded minds of TiTP believe that rather than take responsibility for their own personal choices, people of average weight should be ashamed of themselves for their lack of accommodation. Thin people have all the advantages in the world, and furthermore, they're all "fat shamers" for not being able to incorporate infant elephants into all aspects of human life. Fat shaming is little more than a code word for the lamest form of discrimination I've ever heard of, and it only exists because these hippos conjured a victim out of their dreamscape.

Many point fingers at the Abercrombie & Fitch CEO for publicly discouraging unattractive people from buying his brand's apparel. *Fat shaming* is trying to maintain your company's brand image. *Fat shaming* is designing a roller coaster with restraints that don't come far enough down to click, causing you to fall out in the loop-de-loop. *Fat shaming* is suggesting that you put down the chili cheese fries once in a while and pick up a stick of celery. *I'm trying to help another human being take control of their lives and live longer. Fuck me, right?* Go ahead; add me to the long list of fat shamers. I'll wear that badge with honor. It's not that I don't sympathize with your type 2 diabetes and hypothyroidism. It's the fact that you don't either. I'm not aware of any doctors that prescribe fried chicken and cherry cheesecake as medication for your low blood sugar.

What's really disturbing is the fact that these support groups are gaining in popularity. *This is Thin Privilege* is only the face of an increasingly prominent and perverted trend in society. People would rather promote acceptance of their flaws rather than be persecuted, even if their personal shortcomings are amendable. You can find equal amounts of this hate-filled rhetoric spewing from social media outlets like Facebook and Twitter. The people who share these views form an online clique of sorts, and the more anecdotal horror stories they share amongst themselves, the more these people believe in their confirmation bias. This vocal minority of fat acceptance generalizes the public as enemy #1, and any evidence to counteract their inherently flawed logic is discarded as vitriol. The putrid hyperbole shaped in these threads is contagious, and many filter these jimmy-rustling anecdotes (whether they actually happened or not) through their brains as unequivocal truth.

Along with fat shaming, *thin shaming* has recently become it's own reciprocal force of malevolence. A staggering percentage of the obese think that just because they have been "oppressed" due to their size, it gives them the right to treat others of healthier shape with blatant disrespect. You may have heard about Maria Kang, the mother of three kids who posted a picture on Facebook of her newly toned, postpregnancy body. The caption on the photo: "What's your excuse?" The post sparked a flurry of outrage from fat moms everywhere, who called her a bully, fat shamer, and demanded her apology. Yes, that's right. She should be "sorry" for putting down the donuts and working to improve her self-image. Kelly Ripa, the daytime talk show host, even more recently posted a picture of her abs after trying a new diet program. The comments were equally disgraceful, vilifying her as an anorexic, alcoholic media whore. This is the world we live in, folks. Don't expect the world to be suddenly flowery and great when you've dropped 80 pounds. The value of losing weight is losing the one hater in the world that matters: you. And shedding that personal doubt and building self-confidence is going to make all the difference in your life.

Some of the reactions people have had since my weight loss have been flabbergasting, ranging from whispers of drug abuse to an outright eating disorder. To be honest, they weren't whispers at all. These individuals voiced their profane discontent of my appearance in public and at home, often with others well within earshot.

Personally, I don't take offense to that kind of talk. Not anymore, at least. I'd rather be called a toothpick than a whale any damn day of the week. All these bogus accusations do is reveal the true colors of the people who supposedly "love and support" you, and that nature is often ugly and callous. That said, just because a person falls into a normal weight range doesn't make it any more right to bash on them. Thin people have feelings, too, and those who you feel "oppressed" by might be likely to show more compassion if you show them some in stride. In fact, I think there's a golden rule or something someone came up with a time ago.

I had an anonymous encounter recently with one of these "thin shamers." She wasn't a friend or family member, but a cashier at Sam's Club. This lady was rather large; I'd say in the range of 5' 8", 280 lbs. I wasn't picking up much food this particular trip, mostly beers and Coke Zero. I saw a turkey wrap that looked good as I passed the refrigerated section and threw that in the cart as well. I pulled up to the register and go through the usual, "Hi, how are you?" spiel. She immediately comments on all the beer I have in the cart, asking, "What's wrong? Having a bad night?"

"Nope, just Tuesday," I reply.

I start loading up the cart as she rings up everything, when suddenly I hear it. "Hun, you're going to need more to eat than this."

I had no catalog of responses for this particularly unsolicited comment, so the beta within me just sputtered out, "Yeah, I think I'm good with what I got."

She went on to mention her brothers, elaborating that the turkey wrap I had wouldn't even classify as an appetizer to them. *Well, color me caring!* If similar genetic makeups exist across her siblings, I can only imagine the family feasts of Burger King and Panda Express they share together. Her dissatisfaction with my choice of fare was unwarranted (and quite frankly should be grounds for termination), yet I couldn't help but take a sort of pity on this woman. Her convoluted attitude towards food made her feel superior enough that she had to tell me I was clearly malnourished, yet staring me in the face was the result of what happens as a result of "eating enough." The alcohol comment was weird, too. Why do I have to be depressed to enjoy an adult beverage? I mean, most people I've met wouldn't classify me as a happy-go-lucky guy. But shit, I'm doing quite all right now. Much better than when I looked more like her, I can tell you that. The whole experience that night still gives me heebie-jeebies.

PART II

Transition

Okay, so now you should have, at the very least, a more comprehensive understanding of why it is we become overweight and why it is a growing problem in America and elsewhere in the world. Your struggle with weight is not exclusively your own doing. We, as humans, are very impressionable beings. We like to believe what we're told, trusting that everything will turn out in our best interests. Unfortunately, there remains a consequence for our actions; even those actions encouraged by our own families and loved ones.

As you overcome the obstacles on your path to healthy living, realize that you alone have the power to control how the negative influences around you affect your personal habits and behaviors. Fat is *your* fault, no one else's. The human mind is an incredibly capable machine. It just needs to be programmed to operate with fewer glitches. If you want a computer that works as well as the day you bought it, you have to steer clear of all the pop-ups, spam, and viruses you're exposed to when surfing the web. If you only click one or two malicious ads thrown on your screen, you'll probably be fine.

However, if you install 10 toolbars on your browser and start to believe sexy singles in your area want to fuck you right now, it won't be long before your PC slows to an agonizing crawl.

The body works much in the same fashion. You've probably heard the phrase "treat your body as the temple." While the expression may be derived from the religious texts of yore, this is nonetheless some of the best life advice there is for people of all faiths. If you take care of your body, it will take care of you. Your brain is the apex of that temple. How are you supposed to "think thin" when your neural pathways are clogged with the skin of Church's Chicken? Positive habits can be and are just as addicting as negative ones. Some people run 3 miles everyday for the same reason others smoke a pack of cigarettes a day: it feels good. In the beginning, the runner probably hated the notion of moving or physical exercise whatsoever. Most everyone thinks cigarettes are disgusting at one time or another, yet some choose freely to breathe carcinogens into their lungs without much devoted thought.

When it comes to eating habits, a crash diet is not going to suddenly erase the thoughts of pizza and cheesecake from your long-conditioned mind. Sure, in the short term, you're likely to drop weight like there's no tomorrow. But ask yourself: *could I eat these same foods for the rest of my natural born life?* If the answer is no, then you are all but destined to fail. You have to fall in love, not with food, but with self-control of your appetite. Proper diet is not a punishment, but a reconfiguration. Successful dieters will learn to cherish new and healthier options, while at the same time your favorites of old will fade until you don't even care to seek them out anymore. For me, I learned that mayonnaise isn't the only sauce that tastes good on a sandwich. Diet soda tastes just as good as regular soda if you give it a chance. In fact, the regular stuff is too syrupy for my palette now. The point is, hit the reset on those taste buds, and be open to trying some new things.

The college freshman doesn't expect a degree to be conferred to them after the first week of classes. Your body, in its present state, is that same freshman. Through dedication, perseverance, and learning how this unique machine operates, one can become master of flesh and bone. Crash dieters are the cheaters of health school, who later pay dearly for electing to take shortcuts. I don't have an analogy for student loan debt just yet, but I'm bouncing around a few ideas. Oh yes, I believe dieting school debt is the idea of shelling out for a Bowflex and elliptical machine the day before Thanksgiving. That loan is never forgiven either, a constant reminder that takes up 20 square feet in your living room. The best part of graduating: instead of receiving that drab sheet of paper you get to hang in an expensive frame, you get to share thousands of photos of your new self with your circle of jealous and depressed friends on Facebook!

If you feel up for the challenge, then it's time to brace yourselves, folks. Round 2 of this literary journey is about to begin. Armed with the knowledge of plots, distractions, and schemes aimed at derailing your goals in life, you are now ready to blaze your own trail to health and happiness.

8

Calories Over All

Let's begin with the basics, the foundation. The fundamentals, if you will. *The* absolutely most important figure surrounding anything you ingest and what you should focus your attention primarily on *are*... (drum roll please) calories. Calories are king. Calories are energy. Calories make the body tick. It is the fuel that drives our very existence. Just as the car needs gasoline to drive, the body needs calories to survive.

Calories exist in nearly all the foods we eat. From carrots to cookies, everything we eat adds to our daily caloric intake. Thankfully, our bodies are capable of using and burning these energy morsels by way of our internal metabolism. No matter what we do throughout the day that is physically strenuous, we still burn thousands of calories for nothing more than existing. Sleeping burns calories, breathing burns calories, and sitting on the couch all day burns calories. When you hear of diet programs that promise no-exercise weight loss, they're right. You can be of ideal weight by doing nothing else other than changing your meal plan.

Our bodies are not programmed to naturally look fit and slim. Quite the opposite is true, in fact. Our ancestors were often faced with prolonged bouts of starvation. Occasionally, a very large piece of game or a successful harvest would drop in their laps. Therefore, early humans had to make the most of their windfalls and stretch the benefits of their catch.

I, myself, am often presented with the dilemma of having too much food on hand at one point or another. If it's sitting in my house, chances are that I'm going to eat it, and eat it quick. My brain doesn't know where the next meal is coming from, so I am compelled to stuff myself while food is readily available. When food becomes scarce and the cupboards are bare, I find that the need to engorge myself constantly subsides rather quickly. Our metabolism is designed to store everything it can, much like a camel stores fat in the humps of their backs for a long summer's trek. Unlike dromedaries, however, that critical storage function tends to manifest itself in humans as an unsightly gut.

Maintaining your dream weight is as simple as matching your daily ingestion of calories with the expenditure of your metabolism at that weight. So how do we find the perfect balance of intake to output? This is where technology comes into play. I want you to open up Google on your phone or computer. Type in "BMR Calculator" and click one of the first results to show. What you're looking for is the *Basal Metabolic Rate*, your baseline daily energy expense. From here, you can easily map out the exact amount of calories you need to eat to shred those pounds and make the scale smile. The best way to measure your goal is to enter in your current weight first, then plug in your ideal weight. For me, as a 6'4" 330 lb. early-20s male, my BMR used to be around 2900 calories per day. At my current weight of about 205 lbs., my BMR is only around 2100. If I wanted to gain all the weight back that I lost, I would have to eat 800 calories per day more than I do now. To put this number into perspective: that's an extra cheeseburger and fries, every day, for as long as it takes to pack those pounds back on. Your BMR is the number of calories you would burn if you were sleeping all day long. Even a trip to the mailbox would increase this number significantly. Now, take your newfound BMR and plug it into another online calculator for something called the Harris Benedict Equation. You'll find that even couch potatoes still burn at least 20% in addition to their baseline expenditure.

You can use the difference between your current and

dream BMRs to craft a diet exclusive to your goals. The good news is: if you have 40 lbs. to lose, you may only need to cut out 200 calories a day. The bad news: it's going to take a long time to cut weight if you do it that way. You see, every pound of body fat you carry right now is the equivalent in energy to 3500 calories. Cutting 200 calories a day means you would only lose a pound once every 17 days or so. Most people don't have that kind of time to prep for pool season. The solution is to create calorie deficits that ensure you lose significant amounts of body fat in a relatively short period of time. So, if you would like to lose a pound in a week, you would have to cut roughly 500 calories out of your meals *every day*. This may not sound like much, and it isn't in theory, but keeping to a plan that doesn't cheat this deficit is much easier said than done. A cheeseburger and a milkshake could set your diet back two or three days just because you chose to have lunch at the In-N-Out.

The hardest part of losing weight isn't the diet or exercise. It's math. We're not talking about AP calculus here, either. Addition and subtraction can and should be your biggest allies. Use them. If you have to start multiplying the nutrition facts per serving, you're probably doing it wrong.

I know it may sound cheesy, but if it helps, many have

found success through authoring a daily food journal. Write down everything you put into your body over a 24-hour period, including the sneaky midnight snacks. Writing things on paper wire them into our brains in ways that mental notation, or even typing isn't capable of. If the nutritional information isn't readily available right on the box, bottle, or can of food you're eating, the Internet qualifies as a great substitute. A quick Google search will tell you exactly what perils await within that Outback Steakhouse Bloomin' Onion. Eating at your favorite restaurant or family gathering, it may be difficult to find any kind of ballpark figure about the content of your food. This is no excuse to go overboard. When in doubt about the availability of healthy fare, try to eat *before* going out for celebrations to save yourself valuable time on the treadmill of the future. It's far easier to eat one less slice of cake than it is to run a mile.

    Most commercialized diets have some sort of meal plan to accompany them, which would make the idea of a food diary seem like a moot point. However, these charts and lists only work if you strictly adhere to them, and most plans have at least some foods you don't really care for. I have lived by the regimen of The South Beach Diet, The Atkins Diet, and for a time I even tried the grapefruit diet. I ate one piece of toast for breakfast, one egg for lunch, and stocked my pantry with gallons of pungent citrus juice. Yet no matter what level of enthusiasm I had to begin with, it was only a few weeks at best before my insides shrieked in surrender. It's an incredibly monotonous and shackling way to live life, which is why I suggest you plot your own plan, with foods you can count on sticking to.

Food journals don't work for everybody. It takes a ton of honesty and commitment to document the entirety of things we put into our mouths. The tome that you end up writing might be the most vile and repulsive filth you've read in your entire life (aside from this book, am I right?). The biggest mistake I see people make is not writing down foods they eat because they "don't count." *Onion rings "don't count." It's a vegetable for Pete's sake! That Venti Caramel Frappucino I had this morning with a brownie blended into it doesn't count either, because "drinks don't have calories."*

Liquid calories are the most deceitful and conniving bastards of the nutritional kingdom. Sodas, salad dressings, milkshakes, and nearly any sauce you can think of are taking a viscous dump on you hopes and dreams. Chocked full of sugars and fats, liquid calories are the Trojan Horse of the American diet. Serving little to no nutritional value, these "empty" calories, as they are known, are inherently worthless in satiating appetites. What's worse, the sugar "high" many people experience from glucose-laden drinks draws us in again and again for more. We've been conditioned to think these sweet beasts are normal accompaniments to our entrée of choice. After all, who would think of ordering a dry salad? What's a turkey sandwich without a healthy slathering of garlic aioli? These seemingly innocuous accouterments add up, and they add up fast. If you write it down in a journal, write it *all* down. Don't go soft and get tossed trying to fuck with the liquid.

For many of us, the motivation to work out is a force that is nigh unattainable. For those who do exercise, it's crucial that you don't squander your gains in a post-workout feast. *You hiked Camelback Mountain today? Good on you!* It is a pretty awesome feeling, I must admit. Exercise can be a truly invigorating experience, despite the short-term feelings of discomfort. No pain, no gain though, right? While exercise isn't a necessary part of the weight loss equation, it certainly gives you a huge leg up. Muscles are the bodies' calorie-burning powerhouses. Even when at rest, muscles are utilizing all the available calories we have to stay in a consistently active state. Wonder why Michael Phelps can eat 12,000 calories a day and still have a six-pack? Muscles. For an athlete, failure to eat enough food during the day means taking a hit in performance during competition. These highly tuned human specimens require extreme amounts of fuel to perform at their peak efficiency, much like a Big Rig truck needs hundreds of gallons of fuel for a long haul cross-country. For those of us who would prefer to park our behinds in front of an LCD all day, a little exercise still goes a long way in our continuous battle with the bulge.

If you went ahead and looked up one of the BMR calculators I mentioned earlier, you may have stumbled upon that drop-down list of multipliers based on how active a person you are. In short, exercise increases the amount of calories we can consume while still remaining the same weight. If you decide you want to start running a few miles everyday, your metabolism will increase accordingly. You may burn an extra 1000 calories per week by introducing a simple new exercise plan. Still, over the course of a week, this added effort doesn't even amount to 200 calories of food you could theoretically eat more of per day. It pains me to see people at the gym who view 20 minutes on the elliptical machine as credit enough to treat themselves to a large Dairy Queen Blizzard on the way home. Our westernized culture of instant gratification doesn't coalesce with the substantiated laws of thermodynamics.

Another little morsel of hyperbolic logic I happen upon is that of "eating to avoid starvation mode." It is true that if you don't eat for a certain length of time, your body enters what we call a state of *ketosis*. Ketosis essentially means that your body gets so hungry that it starts devouring itself. If you're not careful, the body not only eats your fat stores for survival, but it will eat muscle as well. The problem with ketosis is that when the next time a big meal comes around, especially with any carbs, your body is literally starving for sustenance and will proceed to pack that food on to your frame as much as physically possible. You can go from slim and starving to Beluga status in the course of an hour. The key, of course, is to regulate the amount of food that we ingest over the span of a day. I'll get more in depth about this later as we discuss some of the proper foods we should eat to avoid these biological hurdles. But for now, know this: six trips a day to McDonalds is not the idea here.

9

The ~~Diet~~ Lifestyle Change

Diet. The word that evokes sentiments of rage, guilt, anxiety, and depression is a fundamental staple of our anatomical vocabulary. To fail is to quit. To win is to struggle. The diet is a regimen, a schedule of sustenance that doesn't meld well with the chaos of life. Diet is a dirty word. Being told to go on one is asking for a response ranging from sneers to snarls. Supermodels swear by it, and others swear of it. Life's a bitch, and then you diet.

A popular figure often quoted in media is that 95% of diets fail. That is, people have regained whatever weight they presumably lost. I have counter theory to this argument, and that is that 95% of diets never really *begin*. To start eating a healthy and more balanced array of foods is just as much of a challenge as anything you can possibly imagine. *Today is the day I turn vegan! Today is the day I start eating organic and gluten free! Today is the day I quit shooting heroin! Today is the day I <insert difficult or impossible task here>.* Skeptics of weight loss exist for the same reason as any other accomplishment's naysayers. If I were to sit at a piano for the first time, put on a wig, and ask you to call me Beethoven, you might have an admonishing laugh as well.

Psychologists have found repeatedly that people get as much satisfaction from *telling* others about their goals as they do actually *achieving* them. After spreading the news from the mountaintops, motivation soon drops, and little is gained other than a few Facebook likes. My advice: *Keep your goals to yourself, and quietly put in the work.* You have to back up your proclamations with real results, or prepare for the wave of backlash that ensues. The proof is in the pudding (or the lack thereof).

You've heard it a thousand times. *A diet is not a diet. It's a lifestyle change!* I'm sure you've become reacquainted with this little quip at many junctures in your life. To be honest, I don't like using conceptual terms to illustrate my deviation in life's grand journey. If you think about weight loss in the abstract, as black and white, the Double Double of the black will always win. No, dieting, as I like to think about it, is simply pushing aside the negative and forgetting the dark side even exists. Dieting doesn't mean that you have to resign yourself to a life filled only with celery sticks and red pepper hummus. You just have to forget the Double Down Sandwich at KFC is an actual thing.

Having a relationship with bad food is like having a relationship with a bad ex. You tell yourself all day that associating yourself with them is bad for your health. They've been lying, cheating, and making you feel like less of a human being for months, maybe even years. However, for a short while at least, they complete you. She's a midnight snack, one text away, and she tastes nothing less than sensational. She fucks like a goddess all night and whispers in your ear that you're all she ever wants in a man.

The sun rises, and you dream of things to come on your way home. The next day, that same old flame posts a picture of herself on Facebook with a guy you've never met, crops you out of all your pictures together, and her relationship status now reads "engaged." The moral of the story: you should have blocked her number and deleted her from your friends list 8 months ago.

Remove your emotional attachment with food, or all you're setting yourself up for is unending heartbreak. Break that shit clean off. Find someone new, someone fresh. If you can't avoid seeing that one toxic woman once in awhile, make it clear that you're just "fuck buddies" now, nothing more. Yes, it will be difficult. Yes, from time to time you'll reminisce of things that once were. But the quickest way to get over your love for pizza will be to get yourself quickly under a juicy Cedar Plank Salmon.

Don't put your goals on hold for tomorrow, because *tomorrow* never comes. Conveniently, it's always a day away. *Free beer… tomorrow!* Your mind likes to play an awful lot of tricks on you, especially just as you're about to fall asleep. As you're lying there, waiting for the sweet embrace of unconsciousness to take hold, suddenly you're imbibed with the motivation to take over the world. *Tomorrow, I'm going to learn Chinese, quit drinking, and have the balls to tell my boss to fuck off!* Needless to say, your alarm goes off in the morning and positively zero of those things come to fruition.

I'm certain that a good percentage of those 95% of diets that fail start out the day before as a full-on binge of all things unholy. This plays into the whole "black and white" mindset of dieting. "Oh my God, I'm never going to have a slice of red velvet cheesecake again! Better go down to the Cheesecake Factory tonight and go out with a bang!" "To celebrate my last night of smoking crack cocaine, I'm going to bang this seven gram rock like Charlie Sheen!"

NO! You lose! Good day, sir! Going cold turkey is as easy or as hard as you make it out to be. If you smoke the rest of your carton of cigarettes the day before you start smoking none, *you're gonna' have a bad time!* When it comes to food, think of blood sugar as a sort of endocrinological nicotine. The highs of today antedate the crashes of tomorrow.

If you're deep in the gutter and have sackfuls of weight to lose, it's better to taper your withdrawal than hack it off at the knee. In fact, cold turkey can spell a death sentence with respects to several addictions. Heroin and alcohol addicts often use prescribed medications to ease the symptoms of withdrawal during detox. Smokers have nicotine patches and gum to fall back on. As far as nutrition goes, your body may or may not be able to handle a sudden slashing of sugar. This could lead to hypoglaecemia or another serious condition. That's why you should always consult a doctor when considering a radical change to your lifestyle, especially when other extraneous ailments are already present. We're not trying to put the "die" in diet here. Ease into your goals. Don't try to run a marathon the day you pick up your first pair of running shoes at Payless.

When people ask how I lost over 100 pounds, they always want to know, "what's your secret?" You've probably read this far into the book just to find out what my secret to weight loss is. Surely, there must be *something*! Okay, fine, I give in. Since you've been patient with me thus far, I'll be delighted to share it with you. The secret... (*dramatic pause*) is that *there is no secret!* I don't attribute my success to The South Beach Diet, The Atkins Diet, The Paleo Diet, or the Weight Watchers plan. I don't stay up late at night planning a breakfast with a half a grapefruit and unbuttered toast and for lunch a hard-boiled egg. I don't have "cheat days" or a list of foods that I refuse to eat. I can't stand in front of you on a pedestal and sell you a dream diet, because no such one exists. If losing weight were as easy as lying on your stomach and eating cupcakes on Thursdays, wouldn't everyone be doing it?

Diet and exercise are not the canned responses most people are looking for in such an inquiry. Furthermore, many can't believe that anyone could possibly achieve something so great without the help of an overly publicized diet plan. When they hear the truth, their responses often turn to the negative, and rumors of every kind begin to spread. Prepare yourself for this, as it is inevitable. Your friends, your family; everyone whom you think supports you will throw accusations of eating disorders and drug use. "It's unfathomable that Marcus could lose all that weight just by eating less! He must be smoking meth now. Yup, meth. If it's not meth, then he's got anorexia for sure! Did you see what he had for lunch? Salmon! He didn't even ask for extra lemon butter sauce! That kid is starving himself!" Don't concern yourself with the critics. Their scorn only thinly veils their own fragile self-image by projecting imaginary problems onto you. When you become the object of envy, you are winning at the game of life. Anyone can have pity taken upon him, but jealousy is earned.

All right, so I've stalled long enough in this chapter already. Let's get into the nitty-gritty of all the foods I stuffed my fat face with to melt that weight right off. For breakfast, I like to start out with a hot, fresh Cinnabon, a full slab of applewood-smoked bacon, French toast sticks with real maple syrup, and a nice tall glass of whole milk. If you're mouth is already beginning to water like a dog's in the drive thru, then *shame on you! You fat fuck! I ought to reach through this page and smack you in your pig snout this very second!* No worries, my friend, we shall exorcise that Pavlovian demon from you in due time.

We, as members of the animal kingdom, have been conditioned to recognize when tasty food is headed our way. Our natural response is to crave and to prepare our bodies for the onslaught of entrée to come. Now, picture in your mind a meal with carrots, grape tomatoes, a turkey burger, and a granny smith apple. The voraciousness of your appetite has perhaps subsided a tad, no? As you progress, these instinctual responses will slowly flip upside down. I'm not saying that you'll stop loving Krispy Kreme donuts in 6 month's time, but it'll be much easier to say no.

I'll be the first to admit that I'm a carnivore at heart. I can't say that if I've had a meal until the flesh of a dead beast swims within me. If you can handle the strictly vegan or vegetarian lifestyle, I bestow oodles of kudos upon you. I cannot. If I arrived in this world with an owner's manuals, it would read: animal protein required. Thankfully, there's more to meat than Polish sausage and 80/20 ground beef. If pressed, I would say my go-to animal entrées are (in general) turkey and chicken. The white meat in poultry tends to have a much higher ratio of protein to fat than red meats, such as beef, bison, or pork. A turkey sandwich or a grilled chicken breast could be one of the healthiest meals you eat all week, and I eat them often. These foods pack an appetite-pounding punch, and fill you up quick. Protein takes longer for bodies to digest than fats or carbohydrates, allowing us to feel fuller for longer periods of time. Don't get me wrong. Red meats have lots of protein too. But when you factor in the added fat of a steak, the baked potato side, and the loaf of free bread at the restaurant table, you're train has derailed for the evening.

Seafood is a great source of lean protein as well. Shrimp, scallops, lobster, crab, and all types of swimmingly fare offer healthy alternatives to the walking dead. Opt for the grilled, steamed, or baked varieties of these dishes, and avoid the deep fried traps of fish 'n chips and the like. Golden butterfly shrimp and coconut shrimp are off limits. The cardinal rule of fish: if you can see the scales, you can beat the scales. Lunch at Long John Silvers will sink you down to Davy Jones' Locker. Steer clear of the copious amounts of melted butter with that lobster tail, and avoid overloading on condiments such as tartar sauce. Low calorie alternatives like cocktail sauce and malt vinegar are your seafood sidekicks.

If feasting on farm animals isn't to your liking, plenty of products made by them have many of the same health benefits. Eggs, especially egg whites, are protein powerhouses. Milk and milk products like yogurt and cottage cheese all help to complete this truly balanced breakfast. Opt for the low-fat or nonfat options when it comes to dairy. Alternative milks like soymilk or almond milk taste near the same (many say *better*) compared to the original. There's sure to be at least one brand to your liking.

As human beings, I realize that not every omnivore

among us can be a barbaric meat eater. If you're keen on living the vegan lifestyle, there are plenty of protein-rich foods that grow right out of the ground. Soybeans, regularly used to make tofu, are very rich in protein. Beans in general are a great source of protein. Peas and lentils are a couple more great options. Hummus, a dish made with chickpeas, is a super healthy dip to use in place of ranch or sour cream. Some other grains, such as quinoa, have about 9 grams of protein per cup. Spinach and kale are killer choices too.

We've been told our whole lives that fruits and vegetables are essential for a healthy diet. Indeed, there are many players in the plant world that have uniquely great things to offer our bodies. Unfortunately, for many years I took "vegetables" to mean French fries and onion rings. Just because it grows on a tree or in a field does not mean it will help you slim down to Chinatown. There is a fair share of landmines to sidestep in the produce aisle.

Take canned fruits, for example. Pears, peaches, and fruit cocktail sure sound like the staples of a straight edge life. They are, too, right up to the point where they get stuffed in a can with a cup full of corn syrup. These once harmless edibles are drowning in liquid sugar, all in the interest of preserving them in your pantry for years on end. Peas, green beans, asparagus, and corn are no better. Despite having fewer calories, canned vegetables and legumes are swimming in their own cauldrons of sodium and preservative-laden broth. The same goes for canned meats and fish, such as SPAM, sardines, or tuna. Pickles and pickled peppers are no better. Even though they're not chocked full of calories, they are full of salt from soaking up the brine they come in. I would avoid the canned food aisle entirely, unless you're one of those doomsday preppers stocking your bomb shelter. Scratch that: don't do it even if you're one of them. Half the people I've seen on that show use the impending end of the world as an excuse to overeat today, especially the ones who cook odious quantities of food before canning it themselves. I guess their logic would be to go down into the bomb shelter with more reserves packed on their body to start with.

Dried fruits can be deceiving in their own respects. Raisins, prunes, and dried apricots are merely condensed versions of their fresh counterparts, retaining every last bit of sugar in the original. It's easy to get carried away when companies are able to fit 400 raisins in a tiny, innocent looking box. Your stomach can fit far more fruit jerky in there when it doesn't have to compete for space with the plant's own natural juices. Therefore, try to eat fruits (and meats, for that matter) in their original, hydrated forms.

While it's important to monitor total sugar intake, especially among diabetics, the next important thing would be to maximize the amount of fiber in your diet. Dietary fiber is a crucial part in any weight loss plan. Fiber, unlike fats, sugars, vitamins, or minerals, is indigestible in humans. We simply "rent" fiber as it passes harmlessly through our gastrointestinal tract. So why on earth would we want to eat it? I like to think of fiber as a sort of "natural filler" in food. Its primary purpose for dieters is to slow digestion, which means that we feel fuller sooner. The slowed digestive process also means that we feel fuller for longer periods of time.

Fiber allows us to eat less now and stave off hunger pangs later. That sounds like a win-win situation to me. Fiber even helps to lower blood cholesterol levels, and it also aids in regulating blood glucose and insulin levels. So what kinds of foods pack a fibrous punch? For starters, berries. A serving of raspberries adds nearly 8 grams of fiber to your diet. Blueberries, strawberries, and blackberries all help too. Beans are full of fiber. Black beans, pinto beans, and kidney beans are some of your best bets. Other winners include artichokes, spinach, carrots, and broccoli.

You may hear that foods like corn, avocados, and

peanuts have tons of fiber too. Be wary of these illusionists! There's a reason they taste so good. While high in fiber, these foods are also high in *fats* and another little thing called *carbohydrates*. We'll get into carbs in a minute. But you have no doubt seen the craze about avocados. Restaurants advertise them as a "superfood", whatever the hell that means. The problem I have with avocados is not that they're unhealthy (far from it, actually), it's that they're usually paired with super-fattening foods like cheeseburgers or tortilla chips. It's little more than a cherry on a milkshake.

Fruits and vegetables can be a pain to have around the house. Fresh greens spoil fast, so unless you consume them in a relatively short period of time, they often end up rotting on the kitchen counter. That just seems like a waste, and it sure doesn't encourage me to fork over more money to stock up again.

Fresh food always tastes the best, but their frozen counterparts make sure you always have some at arm's length. You'd be surprised at just how many of the same fruits and vegetables in the produce department have also made their way to the frozen food aisle. Peas, peppers, berries, onions, and all sorts of other goodies can last for months in your freezer at home, and you only have to use up what you need at any given time. Frozen fruits and vegetables are often stocked with even more nutrients and minerals than fresh counterparts, as these greens are flash frozen at the peak of ripeness instead of maturing on their way from farm to store. As an added bonus, you won't find a salt lick's worth of sodium and preservatives in every bag, like you would in a room temperature can.

Back to the fresh stuff, if sitting down to a full plate of carrots and celery sticks isn't what you would consider appetizing, *juicing* may be your best option. You can find a decent juicer at nearly any store, but don't run out and buy one if you're not positive that juicing is your preferred method of intake. The home juicer falls into the same category of small kitchen appliances as the Ronco chicken rotisserie and the Easy Bake oven, implying they often get used one time and are subsequently banished to the pantry until your next garage sale. You can find prepared health juices such as Naked brand drinks or a V8 to try out before you commit to investing in a juicer. Raw juices are an acquired taste, I promise you that. But like beer, coffee, and cigarettes, many people grow to love their attributes.

The best juices (both nutritionally and taste-wise) will come from home, and the variety of drinks you can whip up is as limited as your imagination. For the best results, try to mix both fruits and vegetables together in the same beverage, erring on the side of more vegetables. The natural sugars in fruits largely overpower the taste of vegetables, making an apple or orange the perfect disguiser of disgust. Just don't go reaching for the raspberry sorbet to sweeten up that borderline-unpalatable beverage. This is not Jamba Juice! Also, please refrain from peeling the raw goods as much as possible. The skins of fruits and veggies are highly fibrous and only serve to aid in your conquest. Try to blend only one serving at a time, as juicing can rapidly deplete the nutritional benefits of the ingredients if left out for any stretch of time (note: this does not mean the drink loses calories if you let it sit in the fridge overnight). Finally, take the time to clean the juicer right after use, so it's ready for the next round later. You don't want to forget about it for a day and then stumble upon a dried, clumpy mess to tend to.

I prefaced the treacherous nature of carbohydrates a bit earlier; so now let's discuss what carbs are and why they can be harmful to weight loss. In a basic sense, sugars *are* carbs. Carbohydrates make up the majority of most people's diets. They are essential nutrients and provide the greatest source of fuel in humans. Have you ever seen photos of Michael Phelps or Lance Armstrong sitting down to dinner the night before a big race? It's pasta, pizza, and cakes all around, often adding up to over 10,000 calories worth. While that might be just another day at the Golden Corral for you and me, these finely tuned athletes require these enormous stores to ensure their muscular endurance for the long day ahead. All things considered, professional competitors may even *lose* weight after stuffing themselves silly, just because they burn calories at a lightning pace.

Carb's greatest strength is also its greatest weakness. Most of us are not planning a grueling and arduous run in the city marathon this week, nor are we training 12 hours a day to become Olympians. With that reality in mind, my recommendation would be to avoid carbs wherever possible. You'll find carbs in many foods you're already familiar with. Candy, chips, soda, and bread all have carbohydrates, and a lot of them. What's worse, these foods are rich in *simple carbohydrates*, a diet-killing monster. Simple carbs are made of just one or two sugar molecules and are the quickest digestible source of energy. You may know quite well what a "sugar rush" feels like. That is the effect of simple carbs hard at work. Sugar injects a dose of high-octane invigoration in the moment. But before you know it, the high has faded, and you're already reaching for your 7th Mountain Dew of the day. These foods spike your blood sugar, diverting your body's attention from burning calories to storing calories. Simple carbs have very little fiber or any real nutritional value (other than calories) and are sitting gelatinously on your thighs in a matter of minutes. These, ladies and gentlemen, are the so-called "empty" calories.

Alas, all hope is not lost on carbs. While it may sound arbitrary, *complex carbohydrates* are the kind that we want to buffer our meal plans with. Complex carbs are strings of connected sugars (sometimes over 10 kinds) that can, in truth, be beneficial for dieters. Complex carbs digest slowly, are better at stabilizing blood sugar, and can be found in many fiber rich foods. Green vegetables, whole grains, beans, lentils, and peas all contain complex forms of carbohydrates. Starchy vegetables like potatoes, corn, and pumpkin have complex carbs too, but unless you're willing to eat these foods without the butter, cheese, or oil, I would suggest staying away from starch. Starchy foods simply have too many calories to contend with. Have you ever heard of another person being described as "corn-fed"? It's not a phrase that people conscious of their weight typically want to hear. Only your dress shirts appreciate a good helping of starch.

It's easy to get caught up in the restrictive thinking of the dieting don'ts. But in actuality, diets should be a new and exciting nutritional adventure. Variety, after all, is the spice of life, and a good diet *should* introduce many new foods into your daily routine. If you think losing weight is all about sitting down to a generic plate of edamame and grape tomatoes, you're already limiting your field of culinary vision. Healthy meals can, in fact, be more flavorful and enticing than their deep fried and sugary counterparts.

I'd like to take this last part of the chapter and tell you about some of the strangely flavorful things I've stumbled upon that have helped in my weight loss goals. I'm just going to come right out and say it. Sushi. Yes, I realize the very word "sushi" conjures unpleasant images in many Americans' thoughts. Who in their right mind would want to indulge in slimy, raw fish? For years, those same images floated within my conscience. It wasn't until about five years ago that I was introduced to the vast and colorful world of Japanese cuisine. It really is an entirely uncharted menu for many people. Imagine your first time stepping into Panda Express, Chipotle, or any ethnic restaurant for that matter. That's what your first time in a sushi joint feels like. The best part that most people don't realize: raw fish is only part of what these restaurants have to offer.

Sushi is merely a term that describes the style in which the rice is cooked, steamed with a vinegar dressing. You're probably familiar with sushi rolls, typically wrapped in sushi rice and seaweed. What you may not know about are some of the various ingredients you can find within: cooked crab, shrimp, avocado, and even cream cheese. Yes, some sushi rolls have cheese. Does it sound a bit more appetizing already? Well, perhaps the best thing about sushi is how light a meal can be on your body. A full sushi roll (cut into 8 slices) may contain just 300 calories all put together. Point blank: it's hard to go overboard unless you're really trying. I always leave a sushi place stuffed to the gills, with only a feeling of regret left unfulfilled.

Once you build up your confidence, I highly encourage you to try some of the raw fish rolls. Sushi chefs are generally very proud and dedicated to their craft, and raw fish poses few health risks compared to other meats. *It's fucking delicious, to boot.* The tuna, salmon, and eel rolls are some of the more common offerings. For the truly courageous, you can even try sashimi, which is just raw, sliced fish served up neat. From being a lifelong skeptic to now a fanatic, the only thing I regret about sushi is not trying it earlier. I can't recommend it enough for new and experienced dieters. The only caveats I have here are to avoid any menu item that has "tempura" in front of it. These items are battered and deep-fried. Cream cheese is also not especially healthy, only adding excess calories to the mix. Keep from drowning rolls in the soy sauce, spicy mayo, or eel sauce too. Wasabi is your safe, spicy friend.

Other Asian eateries are also great bets. Thai, Vietnamese, or Indian restaurants all have their own array of unique and exotic fare. There's a reason Asian nations still have some of the lowest instances of obesity in the world. Many, if not most dishes come with a plentiful serving of vegetables, enhanced with savory sauces that you may soon come to know as your favorites.

Unfortunately, while you may have developed a newfound affinity for eastern cuisine, it's likely that your friends and family haven't shared the same enthusiasm. Therefore, your next course of action would be to find the items on the menu of your favorite restaurants that correlate well with your goals. Gloss over the bestselling, gluttonous options and snipe out the healthy offerings. They may be further back on the menu, or buried under a mountain of fried and fattening options, but most restaurants do cater (at least somewhat) to thin thinking patrons. Remember, you only need to find one good option. Pluck that dish out, and make it your new favorite friend. Salmon is one of my "can't go wrong" treasures, so long as it isn't swimming in buttery sauces or cheese. You can find halibut and other healthy fish entrées at nearly any steakhouse or seafood restaurant, too. At the deli or sub shop, turkey sandwiches are your tried and true friends. If they're available, opt for the tortilla wrapped versions (or even bowl versions) of your favorite hoagie. You'll cut a mountain of carbs and calories right out, while still getting your face on all the goods inside.

I'm not a huge salad fan myself, but a properly prepared bowl of greens is the bread and butter of diet plans (figuratively speaking). I find it simply appalling, though, that restaurants can add so many unhealthy accompaniments to the lettuce and still call it a "salad". Berries, nuts, cheeses, meat, and dressings all tip the salad scales from healthy fare to honeypot. Indeed, I've seen salads on restaurant menus that contain the same amount of calories as two Big Macs! Ditch the feta, hold the bacon, and ask for dressing on the side.

Salad dressing is the final nail in the crouton coffin. Often chocked full of fats and sugars, pouring heaps of dressing on your salad is like taking a diarrhetic dump on your dreams. Apologies for the imagery, but I'd like to clear up some misconceptions about what constitutes an appropriate salad topping. Any sauce or dressing that has a creamy or white color to it is inherently bad. We're talking about Caesar, ranch, blue cheese, and thousand island types. Have you looked at the back of any of these bottles? A single serving, which is often a measly 2 tablespoons, can have over 100 calories in it. To put that into perspective, 2 tablespoons of dressing covers about six leaves in a salad. The portions I see many people drizzling on their greens suggest that over 500 calories are added in dressing alone. Folks, that's a cheeseburger in a cup. You're far better off choosing oil-based dressings such as vinaigrettes or honey mustard. Either way, go light on the pour. Every square inch of salad does not need to be moist like the morning dew.

The same applies for most other foods and their sauce cohorts. Ideally, food should taste so good that no sauce is required. But, as a sauce enthusiast myself, I know this is not always the case. The key is to substitute your favorite sauces with healthier options. If you can't eat fish sticks without dunking them in tartar sauce, try ketchup for a change. Yes, ketchup. I was skeptical at first too, but even if it's not your favorite right now, tastes change. Tomato-based condiments like ketchup, barbecue sauce, and cocktail sauce are far better options than mayonnaise-based types like tartar sauce. If you don't like ketchup on fish, try malt vinegar, another great option. Spread mustard instead of mayo on your favorite sandwich. That's what lifestyle change is all about. It's adding variety to the monotony. Switching sauces could save you hundreds of calories per meal, and those savings will add up fast.

It's also time to cut the cheese (literally). It may sound blasphemous, but that thin slice of cheese on your sandwich is little more than a calcium-filled slab of fat. Think of all the foods you like to put cheese on. Pasta, salads, sandwiches, steaks, and the list goes on and on. All these foods work perfectly on their own, minus any curds to subsidize their flavor. We (as Americans especially) have been trained to think that cheese belongs in every nook and cranny we can fill it with. When I go to Subway and order a sandwich, the third question after bread and meat is, "What kind of cheese do you want?" When I respond with "none," you should see the look of shock on the sandwich artists' faces. It's like I gutted a puppy in front of them and smeared the entrails all over the sneeze guard. The thought of a cheese-less sub is incomprehensible to many, yet it's not too hard to understand why. Take a look at what the people in front of you in line are ordering. When you see these other lost souls demanding double-meat, double-cheese, chicken bacon ranch sandwiches on cheesy jalapeno bread, it's easy to see why healthcare costs in this country are soaring to the moon. Trust me. Skip the cheese, pile on the veggies and honey mustard, and call it a win. You can get double veggies at no extra cost. I promise you won't even miss the provolone.

Butter is the same battle. Try to enjoy a bowl of rice or a baked potato without butter, and face the vilification of your fellow man. Everyone knows margarine is bad. You've probably seen the segments on the news or heard from your personal doctor that margarine clogs your arteries faster than the I-10 during rush hour. The consensus is uncontested. Butter is *better*. But that doesn't mean butter is good either. You'll hear people rave on about how a pat of butter only has 36 calories. *36 calories, wow! I should butter every damn thing on my plate!* What the experts neglect to tell you is how tiny a "pat" of butter really is. A pat of butter is less than 1 tablespoon of butter. That's not even half a notch on the butter stick ruler. It's just not worth it. There's a new craze about "grass-fed" butter you may have heard some things about. It's supposed to be chocked full of nutrients that other processed butters lack. Just be keen and use your best instincts. Butter and other butter-like products will have you dancing with the devil three more songs than you intended to.

Now, let's talk about some of the foods that give the "appearance" of being healthy. It's immensely popular for marketers in our society to print health benefits in big bold font on whatever box of food they're selling. Companies team up with well-known diet authorities like Atkins, Weight Watchers, or The South Beach Diet in pushing their "healthy" foods from their fridge to yours. Microwaved, ready-to-eat meals make it a breeze to eat like a champion, or so you would think. First of all, the sizes of these entrées make a Happy Meal look like a three-course feast. You wouldn't have a tough time at all fitting 100 boxes of Lean Cuisine in your freezer, and many indeed do just that. The one thing they have going for them is portion control. Most boxes contain less than 500 calories. That's a great start, but I have a hard time personally stomaching the dish in its vanilla form. Many of these meals are unequivocally tasteless, and more often than not I'm reaching for the salt, Parmesan cheese, and Tobasco sauce to pry my senses from despair. What surprises me most is the quantity of latent sodium and preservatives present in these bland meals. A Smart Ones meal could cap out your whole day's sodium intake limit without so much as a hint of tangible spice in return.

In weight loss, putting a cap on the amount of sodium in our bodies can be just as important as counting calories. Sodium is naturally present in most foods, but most of our consumption comes from in the use of table salt. It's important, chiefly among those with high blood pressure, to reduce the amount of salt in our diets as much as we can. Lowering the amount of sodium we consume has one major benefit aside from aiding those with hypertension. Water retention, or "water weight" as many refer to it as, is a huge factor contributing to that number on the scale (and that frown in the mirror). Rather than flushing water out by natural means, our bodies will store water in equilibrium to the amount of sodium currently sitting within us. More salt means more water, meaning more weight. Less salt, less water, and well… you get the picture.

Fighting water retention is a two-front battle. Obviously, passing on the salt shaker and eating less salty foods is the ideal game plan. But exercise, and sweating in general, will help rid the body of excess NaCl also. A nice session in a steamy sauna can also help purge the body of accumulated liquids. The first week or so of losing weight is primarily where this water is "melting off," so don't think that you're going to continue losing 10 pounds every week going forward. Body fat can't simply be "flushed" out the way water can.

Skipping the salt doesn't have to be a bother, either. Many brands offer salt substitutes containing Potassium Chloride, a molecular cousin to table salt. The recommended daily allowance of KCl in humans is much higher than that of regular salt, yet most people consume less. Potassium also doesn't retain water like sodium does, so shake away. It's not an acceptable alternative for everyone, however. People who take certain medications or already have conditions such as renal failure, heart failure, or diabetes should consult with a doctor before using salt substitutes.

You'll notice very soon the effects of reducing sodium in the diet, namely the disappearance of symptoms such as bloat. That water weight is going to pour away in a flash. Your heart and blood pressure are also going to thank you for the change of habit. I'm sure you know at least a few people who shower their food in salt before even giving it a taste, no matter what the entrée is. What may be surprising is that much of our food sharply lacking in flavor is not due to missing salt. It's missing acid, a problem that can be quickly remedied with your choice of citrus fruit. Try adding lime juice to your next grilled chicken, and unlock the sleeping fowl within. Lemon juice goes great on tacos, burritos, and seafood too. Experiment with citrus, and see how much additional salt you really need.

I can't possibly cover all the hypothetical meal combos you are going to encounter in the day-to-day life. All I can advise is that you use your best judgment. When in doubt, stick with what you know. There's no shame in making chicken fajitas for lunch and then finding yourself eating the same thing at Chili's for dinner. Your metabolism isn't a whiny toddler dragging you to every ride at the amusement park. Don't let your tongue be. Just because everyone else at the table is feasting on soups, salads, and appetizers before the main course doesn't mean you're obligated to participate. If you really want to lose you're appetite, bring your food journal to the Macaroni Grill next time. You might get sick as the calorie count hits four digits before your Penne Rustica even hits the table.

    It should be easier to manage a diet at the restaurant than anywhere else, really. The waiters and waitresses are obligated to bring you whatever you ask for. Don't ask for your death warrant and a pen to sign it with. See if they offer half-orders or a senior menu, so you won't end up with a mound of food left when the check comes (your party will appreciate the lesser expense too).

    Eating at home is another matter entirely, of course, and you may rarely get to decide what is ending up on your plate for dinner. If you're not in charge of grocery shopping for your household now, it's high time to start. You'll at least have a tad more authority on what food comes through the front door. If at all possible, shop for what the house demands and then shop for yourself. You shouldn't have many others fighting over the turkey wraps when the take-and-bake pizza is sitting right next to them. Respect the fact that other people in the house have differing opinions on what it means to diet, but proceed to remove those temptations from your field of view. To take it a step further still, set up a box in the fridge with your name on it. Or, if you're lucky enough to have a second fridge, put your edibles in there. Do what you have to do to withdraw yourself from the source of your unhappiness.

    I don't have to remind you that junk food is a tantalizing temptress, but what about drinks? We all enjoy a nice, tasty beverage on the side to wash down our meals. More importantly, our bodies require liquid refreshment at a rate that far exceeds our need for foodstuffs. Humans can live for roughly three weeks without any nutritional sustenance, but we can die of dehydration in only three days. Drinks can be mixed, shaken, and stirred in an infinitely various number of ways, and many are the most deceitful facets of your diet. It's near impossible to judge the calorie content of a drink simply by looking at it, and your body has a hard time telling the brain when you're full on liquids. The key, just as with food, is to read the labels or search online about the contents within your elixir of choice.

Water is the undisputed king of hydration. Our ancestors have been drinking water since the beginning of time, and it is by far the purest substance we put into our bodies. Zero calories, zero regrets. I'm sure you've heard the advice to drink eight glasses of water a day. While not based on any real science, it's a pretty good rule to follow. That equates to a half-gallon of water, more than you're probably accustomed to. However, the benefits of staying fully hydrated are several-fold. All of your mind and body processes work at full capacity when they have enough water to support their operation. Nutrients can be carried more efficiently to all parts of the body, especially to the outer reaches of your limbs and skin. If you have really dry, rough skin, it could be a direct result of dehydration.

Initial weight loss is largely due to flushing the excess water from the body, so it is vital that you replenish these stores. Remember, water retention is not caused by the overconsumption of water, but by sodium. You might lose 20 pounds of water in the first week or so, but failing to rehydrate could result in a slowing down of the concurrently ongoing fat-burning process. Low water levels also contribute directly to low blood volume in your cardiovascular system.

This causes a reduction in the oxygen available to your muscles and can leave you unnecessarily fatigued. Water also lubricates the joints and reduces the soreness you feel in the muscles and joints post-workout.

Water doesn't just come in a tall glass either. Water is present in nearly all the food we eat, which is both a good and a bad thing. Occasionally you may think you're hungry, but really it's just your body craving more water. Eating can help satiate this thirst, but the cost of quenching means ingesting excess calories that you were probably better off without. If you're not sure whether you're hungry or thirsty, drink a glass of water first to find out. Drinking water before every meal also fills the stomach, allowing you to eat less at mealtime while still feeling full. Think of it as a coupon for 20% off your next chin.

Let's face it, though. Water is boring. Water only tastes good after a good workout or a long night out drinking. Many of us would generally prefer a glass of tea, soda, juice, or coffee instead. And this is where the diet goes to straight to hell. There are healthy versions of all these drinks too, so look out for some of the telltale signs.

A nice hot cup of tea can brighten anyone's day. In its

most rudimentary form, tea is little more than the extract of leaves soaked in boiling water. This, in itself, is an incredibly healthy beverage. It makes sense that all teas would be good for us then, right? Well, the problem with many teas today is the addition of that little thing called sugar. Sweet teas abound in restaurants and on grocery store shelves. Just because it's a non-carbonated drink with the word "tea" in it doesn't make it any better than other drink options. When you're on the prowl, opt for the unsweetened varieties of your choice flavors.

    A can of sweetened tea could have just as many calories as your favorite soda. Coca-Cola and other carbonated beverage manufacturers are facing harsh criticism today for their part in causing a worldwide obesity epidemic. If you counted out the grams of sugar in just one 12-ounce can you might rethink ever picking up that syrupy nectar again. What's worse, many people encourage the use of full-calorie sodas over their diet counterparts. Why? It's all about that cancer-causing, brain-killing compound called aspartame, of course. There's nothing wrong with sugar or high fructose corn syrup, because those ingredients are "all natural". *Please. You know what else is all natural? Arsenic, cyanide, and asbestos.* The FDA has asserted time and again that aspartame is, in truth, one of the most heavily tested substances they're ever evaluated. The FDA has concluded that there's no danger to humans whatsoever with regards to diet drinks. So, chug away on that Coke Zero and congratulate yourself for saving nearly 150 calorie's worth of sugar in every can.

More so than the pseudoscience, many have the need to detest diet sodas simply for their taste. It "tastes" unnatural, therefore it must be bad. Let me tell you something. I had the same line of thinking for many, many years. I couldn't stand the taste of a Diet Coke. However, I would drink a 12-pack of the Classic stuff any day of the week. 12 x 140 calories is 1680, or about the average daily caloric intake recommended for many adults. It's easy for me to see now why that stubborn weight just wouldn't come off! Fast-forward to today, and the opposite is true as far as tastes go. Coca-Cola is far too heavy for my liking. I can *feel* how syrupy it is as it sloshes around, not to mention the sugary film it leaves behind all over the mouth and throat. It is most unpleasant, indeed.

Some research suggests that diet sodas may actually boost appetites, leading to a net gain of calories overall. I'm not too sure of that myself. I can only offer my anecdotal experience, but diet soda has never caused me to eat anything I wasn't planning on devouring already. I would shy away from soda in a few situations, however. The Phosphoric acid, caffeine, and carbonation in soda hinders calcium uptake in bones, which could accelerate osteoporosis or slow the healing process in broken bones. Carbonated water can also deprive your muscles of oxygen, which will in turn affect exercise. Given the choice, though, pick diet as often as you can. Would you rather risk a minuscule chance of cancer, or face the very real prospect of type-2 diabetes and cardiovascular disease?

Fruit juices are even more bamboozling than teas. Have you ever had a glass of orange juice, lemon juice, or grapefruit juice freshly squeezed from the plant itself? It's bitter and a bit lacking in the flavor department. So what makes these fruit favorites taste so great? Correct again: sugar. Take a gander at the fine print on the labels, and soon you'll find how much actual cranberry juice is in that cranberry juice cocktail. Some "juices" contain only 5% (or even less) real fruit juice. It's very easy for companies to replicate the taste of fruits with artificial flavoring, plus they realize you won't know the difference after they add a cupful or two of sugar to the mix. Simply Lemonade? Simply Limeade? How about simply water, a hint of lime, and a cup of sugar. That smoothie you love from Jamba Juice is playing the same game, adding profane amounts of sherbet, peanut butter, and chocolate to your health fix. The fact is, you're gong to have to scour the aisles high and low for 100% juice, or squeeze it yourself at home.

Even 100% juice from the store lacks one of the core components that makes eating the whole fruit a better option still: fiber.

The deacon of diabetes is indubitably the concoction crafted by your favorite hometown barista. Coffee, as it is otherwise known, has a staggering array of customization options available to you. It comes as no surprise that few of these alchemical elixirs can be categorized as "diet-friendly." Espressos, macchiatos, cappuccinos, frappucinos, and lattes all leave the brew spout as benign beverages, but that just doesn't coalesce well when it comes to our finicky preferences. After all, coffee by itself is a distinctively bitter drink, an acquired taste to many. Rather than stomach the virgin nature of the black beast, millions prefer to make the ground bean a visitor to the party rather than the main attraction. Cream, sugar, half and half, flavored syrups, and even alcohol are regular additions to the morning cup of joe. And because we like our coffees to be sweet, and not bitter, unholy amounts of these cup condiments are fundamental in ridding all but a hint of the fresh roast's flavor.

I'm just going to call this one as I see it. Coffee is worse than soda. At least most people realize that soda is unhealthy for you. Coffee has yet to reach that level of awareness, yet some of the most popular coffee options in America are more akin to a milkshake than a brown tea. Take, for instance, the worship-worthy Caramel Frappucino from Starbucks. Compared to a 140 calorie, 12-ounce can of Classic Coke, a Frappucino of the same size has 300 calories in it. *Talk about a 2 for 1!* For some gluttonous goons, that coffee still isn't sweet enough. No, they have to go and do the unthinkable. See those brownies in the display case that Starbucks sells? People ask for those to get blended, *in their coffee*! It's easy to see, if you're a bean fiend, why trips to the corner cafe every day could shortly spell dire consequences. Do yourself a favor and drink it black, or add sugar substitutes like stevia and call it a day.

Coffee is a great way to get through the day, but as the sun sets, I prefer to have a *real* drink myself. Nothing helps the mind forget the woes of yesterday and the stresses of tomorrow like a good, stiff alcoholic beverage. Alcohol is the great bonding agent of the human race, bringing together family and friends like no other drug can. Sure, there's weed too, but how many of you can honestly say you've smoked with your mother, father, aunts, cousins, and brother-in-law? No, *alcohol* is universal.

It's hard to turn down a drink at social gatherings, which is precisely why I rarely do. Unless I have plans to drive later, why not indulge a little bit? A shot here, a beer there, and suddenly all the folks that you avoid 360 days of the year are much more tolerable to be company around. But watch out. There's likely someone sitting at the table or barstool next to you that has developed the so-called "beer gut" over the years you've known them. Amassed by anatomically hoarding several 30 packs of Budweiser and Pabst Blue Ribbon each week for the past 15 years, the beer belly guy is always bringing his own keg to the party. We'd all like to not be "that guy", so how is it that we can slim down and at the same time get wasted?

Unfortunately, alcohol is one of the very few drinks where there is no non-caloric substitute. Alcohol (ethanol, more specifically) is derived from sugar. No amount of light beers or vodka chillers is going to save you from this fact. That being said, some drinks are better for the gut than others, and they're relatively easy to single out.

Let's start with the beers. Nothing is more gentlemanly than sitting down to an ice-cold craft brew after a long day. The flavors that some of these microbreweries put out today are extraordinary, to say the least. Each beer's malted barley and hops meld together to forge a refreshment that is the stuff of legends. Beer has been an integral part of human culture for many millennia, and it shows no sign of stopping now. So what kinds of beers are better for us than others?

Well, it depends. Light beers and heavy beers alike have about the same proportion of calories to alcohol by volume. You may think you're getting off easy by drinking a 64 calorie beer, but that 2.5% abv beer is worth roughly one-third of it's weight in alcohol content compared to it's heavy equivalent. If you're the type that likes to drink to get drunk, your money is going further every time by opting for the heavy beer. However, if you're the social drinker who just wants to have a beer in your hand for the next time someone shouts a toast, the light beer is your better bet. You won't be nearly as drunk as your friends, but you also won't have to work off that heavy beer weight.

This doesn't necessarily explain the beer belly, though. Sure, pounding down 12 beers in a night at 150 calories a pop is going to set you goals back a bit. What really gets the waist expanding, though, is what you choose to eat throughout those drinking hours. As we ingest alcohol, our livers begin to work overtime to burn and metabolize the poison (as it sees it), neglecting other bodily processes like fat burning. Insulin is also released in excess during drinking, which portends low blood sugar. How do our brains tell us to fix this? *Eat more carbs. Reach for that bowl of pretzels at the table. Order that plate of 7-layer nachos and hot wings.* How many times have you eaten a full dinner before you started drinking, only to order a large pizza and breadsticks at 1 AM? Thank your blood sugar. And now that your liver is in a fragile state, that additional food is not even going to be digested remotely properly, ending up on your frame in all the wrong places. You pass out and wake up in the morning feeling like death incarnate. Know what would make that growling stomach feel better, though? Let's find that box of pancakes in the pantry and fry up some bacon. Hang. Over. Cured. Rinse and repeat at least three or four times a week, and voila! You've gestated yourself a beer baby.

Beer isn't everyone's drink of choice, we know. Many prefer the sting of good, hard liquor. Spirits, thankfully, have a few benefits that make it a better option than beer for regular drinking. Beer, no matter how light or heavy, contains carbs as part of the brewing process. These carbs are mostly simple sugars and serve no real nutritional value. Beer does have some B Vitamins and actually about a gram of soluble fiber, but carbs are an enemy that we'd rather live without. Hard liquor contains *zero* carbs. Rum, vodka, gin, and whiskey eliminate carbs through distilling, leaving behind a more pure and concentrated product. Discarding the carbs also leaves behind some of the latent calories you'll find in beer. Comparing a beer to an 80 proof (40% abv) shot of liquor, that shot has about 100 calories, or roughly two-thirds the amount of a similar serving of full-bodied ale.

Tipping back shot after shot all night can quickly turn a good evening into a ruinous affair, so many prefer to mix cocktails instead. Mixing a cocktail takes that one shot and buffers it out over time, giving you the chance to enjoy that straight liquor while others at your table sip on whatever they're having. Be careful, though. The mixers you add to your liquor of choice are what separate the fat from the fit. Margaritas, daiquiris, piña coladas, and Long Island Iced Teas are some of the more popular drinks you'll find at the bar. These are the types of drinks you want to shun away from. The flavorings that make these drinks so delectable are coincidently chocked full of sugars, turning one carefree shot into a rum Frappucino.

What you really want to do to complete that cocktail is add some of the low calorie drinks I mentioned earlier. Do what I do and mix Jack Daniels with a Coke Zero. Make a rum iced tea, but keep that tea unsweetened, of course. You could also take Captain Morgan, Diet Coke, and lime and make yourself a bona fide Cuba Libre. Find sugar free syrups like

Torani and make your own vanilla raspberry vodka. Plan on walking around in the sun or going to the beach for the day? Gatorade and vodka go hand in hand to make Fade-orade, an electrolyte-packed punch keeping you hydrated and wasted at the same time! Experiment with your own recipes at home and arm yourself with an arsenal of mixology for when you're out for a night on the town.

I'll leave the watering hole here with a little bonus, and this last category can be nearly as bad for you for the same reasons as the coffee mentioned earlier. *Drum roll, please*: the energy drinks. I'm talking about Gatorades, Powerades, Monsters, Rock Stars, Red Bulls, and whatever else gets you amped up like a rattlesnake on PCP. You've seen the commercials, billboards, and promotions everywhere you go. Your favorite sports star chugs electrolytes and sweats purple before making the buzzer beater. *Drink me, and become a superstar!* That's the message being sold to millions of people who look up to these heroes of the field and court.

The drink itself can be very beneficial to athletic types, as it not only fulfills the body's need for water, but also helps to retain fluids and replenish electrolytes lost through sweat. That's why I mentioned the Fade-orade earlier, because a few hours walking the pier or swimming in the ocean would be rather taxing on the body.

For the majority of us couch-warmers, though, water is plenty sufficient to meet our hydration needs. If you feel like you can't get through the day without a mind-blowing dose of jittery goodness, reach instead for the little energy shots on the counter at the convenience store. 5-Hour Energy and other similar products have near zero calories and often don't have the crash potential of their sugary rivals. You'll still be blasting away those TPS reports before noontime.

Since we're on the topic of energy drinks, I'll take a minute here to steer you clear of their edible counterparts: energy bars. You know there's something seriously wrong when you can find chocolate candy bars next to the Tylenol at the grocery store. Snickers Marathon, Power Bars, and Slim Fast bars are nothing but candy in disguise. There are a few healthy exceptions that you may find to be a great snack, but as a general rule, don't eat food that comes in bar form. That's bad form.

Alas, I've broached but a morsel of the good and evil counterparts in the diet of the average American. There are endless trials and tribulations waiting as you continue on your culinary journey. However, what I've covered thus far is enough for you to take back control of your appetite and equip you with the knowledge to mind what you put into your body. You must now take the reigns from here. Become the auditor of food and drink, the presiding judge of the food court. When in doubt, chuck it out. There's no shame in throwing away a frozen pizza or that leftover cake when you know it contributes directly to your grief. The opportunities you'll gain by having a stronger sense of self-worth and pride are far more valuable than the uneaten DiGiorno supreme you paid for at Target.

I highly encourage you to head directly into the next chapter, one in which I'll be discussing how exercise fits its way into our health's equation. For those of you who don't plan on exercising anything but your eye muscles today, just skip down to the one after. It will always be here if you change your mind. I realize the very thought of working out can be depressing in itself, so I don't want to overload a whole lot of negative, helpless, or hopeless feelings into your brain right now. Some psychologists might argue that mentioning the notion alone means I already have. *Damn!* Well, now it seems you have no choice but to turn to the next page. That or put the book down in an act of silent protest. *But what the hell did I ever do to deserve that kind of treatment?* I promise this next section won't hurt… too much.

10

Working Out or: How I Learned to Stop Worrying and Love the Burn

Exercise is purely optional when it comes to weight loss. That's just science. You can lose 20 pounds or 200 pounds just by cutting out the excess in your diet. That being said, what you won't get with a diet alone is *in shape*. You want to look like The Rock or Arnold Schwarzenegger? Get lifting, son. Slimming down is one thing, but bulking up in the right places is another entirely. Don't fret about building super-sized biceps just yet, though. If you're overweight, your best bet is to slim down first, and worry about gains later.

What bothers a lot of people about losing weight is the prospect of becoming "skinny-fat." You can lose all the weight you want, but you may still end up with that little extra ponch hanging out front that nobody cares for. Some people would rather be big, fat, and intimidating than risk being small and frail. Make no mistake, after losing the weight that I did, I much prefer skinny-fat over fat-fat any day of the week.

However, just because you hit your goal weight doesn't mean the journey's ended. Skinny people have body image issues as well.

Exercise has many benefits other than just "getting ripped." For one, exercise increases your metabolism, which can aid in accelerating weight loss. Muscles burn significantly more calories per pound than your fat stores, and that's around the clock. They bigger they are, the more fuel they require to maintain their girth. Muscles thrive off of protein, especially post-workout. After hitting the weight bench, make sure you follow it up with a good protein shake, eggs, or a turkey sandwich. Workouts break down the fibers in muscles, so they actually become weaker immediately afterwards. It's important that they get the nutrition required to build back stronger than they were before. Think of your post-workout meal as a reward for a job well done, but don't eat more than any other time of day. You haven't "earned" a cheeseburger or an extra breast of fried chicken.

Bodybuilders have to eat (a lot). We overweight folks have a leg up when it comes to gaining weight, it's just the manner in which we do it that's a bit lacking in its execution. For this reason, losing weight should take precedence before trying to make significant muscle gains. It's very difficult to cut fat and build muscle simultaneously, for the reason that losing requires cutting calories while the other entails adding. But don't think exercising won't help until you've reached your goal weight. Every little bit helps. Just stay consistent and don't be let down when you're hard work isn't immediately translating into a Hurculean frame. You'll still be getting stronger, and you'll already be far ahead of the pack when any kind of continuing training plan is put into place.

Spending time at the gym has one very important, yet often-overlooked benefit. Aside from your muscles, working your body lends itself to boosting your *brainpower*. Anxiety and depression are two common conditions associated with being overweight, and those swirling vessels of negative thought contribute much to the addiction of food. But have you ever noticed the glow that some people have when they start a workout regimen, even those who are still overweight? Most likely, that vivaciousness is attributable to the release of endorphins the brain produces during and after time at the gym. These endorphins make us feel more confident and better about ourselves as a whole, and how we feel on the inside most definitely reflects on the people around us. Before long, you'll want to chase that endorphin high and won't feel right without a good pump in the morning.

So what's the first step towards this utopian ideal of feeling and looking better? Well, since we've got a lot of weight to lose, implementing a cardio routine into our day is going to net us the most progress. These exercises are useful to gym rats in the "cutting" stage, when they're trying to lose fat and increase muscle definition. That's what we want to achieve, because though it may not look like it, we all have show-worthy abs hiding under that gelatinous suit. Implementing cardio can be as simple as an early morning walk around the block or taking the stairs at the mall instead of the elevator. Running, swimming, biking, and time on the elliptical machine are also great tools for slimming down the body.

These exercises can be as easy or as difficult as you make them out to be. If you're overweight or clinically obese, it's not uncommon for you to be suffering from knee and/or back problems. This is entirely okay. Don't push yourself to the point where you injure what capacities you do have. That doesn't mean you get to use your present ailments as an excuse to do nothing. I promise you, most of these afflictions will be eliminated entirely or significantly alleviated in due time. Baby steps: that's all you have to strive for. For starters, a good hop in the pool will work magic. Swimming takes a ton of the strain off your joints, being arguably one of the lowest-impact exercises around. As a bonus, swimming is one of the most effective cardio exercises out there, rivaling jogging and cycling. Spend an hour in the pool everyday, if you have one at your disposal. Build up the amount of laps you swim until you start blending in with the fish. Spend only enough time in the shallow end to turn laps. If you're a bit self-conscious in public of all the splashing around, tread water. Floating under your own power in the deep end *is* an exercise, believe it or not. Just don't let me see you leaving the water without a good set of prunes on your fingertips.

I understand that not all of us have access to aquatic recreation, so work with what you do have. If you're having a tough enough time as it is getting around the house, I would start weight loss through diet alone. When you're back on your feet (so to speak), ease your way into a nice stroll through the neighborhood, or start parking in the back of the lot at Walmart. If you have a gym nearby, try some other low-impact cardio equipment like the elliptical or the stationary bike. And just like the couch you're sitting on, you can still watch TV and play video games doing both of these. What more could you ask for?

The transition from beached whale to cardio bunny is not a short trek by any means. Everyone would like to be able to finish a marathon at some point their lives, but running or jogging I would reserve for intermediate and advanced dieters only. The strain of these high-impact workouts could irreversibly damage your body, from your ankles up to your spine. Try to reach at least 50% of your weight loss goal before adding a light jog to your routine. It's imperative that you find a pair of shoes that help your feet help you. Orthotic soles from certain specialized brands help combat issues like flatfeet or high arches. The best way to find out what works for you is to visit a running store, or ask your foot doctor. Ease into these high velocity workouts, and soon they will pay off in spades.

    Lift up your shirt and look down at your belly right now. If you're proud of what you see, I'm not sure why you've kept reading this far. You've either been doing these things I've mentioned for months already, or you're in some level of denial that this book won't help. Science has shown that's it's impossible to target weight loss to any specific problem area, and that area for most people is in the abdominal region. If you want to get rid of that unshapely gut, but you have thighs of thunder to go with it, it's going to take awhile. Any weight lost is going to be proportionally shed in both of these areas. Shed 10 pounds overall, and you're gut may only lose 3. Your body doesn't care what the mirror thinks you should lose.

Think of your torso like the core of an onion, with fat being the outer layers. As you gain fat, layers are piled up from the inside out, with fat eventually reaching to your outermost limbs. When you lose fat, that process is reversed in the same order. If you packed on a second chin after you filled out the man boobs, the chin will be the first to go.

Peeling back these layers can take a significant amount of time. Thankfully, there are steps we can take to help along these unsightly areas, or at least make them appear better in the interim. Cardio exercises are the kings of cutting fat, but to really show off those "glamour" muscles, *weight training* is your best friend.

Just as with any cardio routine, you want to start small with your ambitions in the weight room. You're not going to walk into the gym and immediately start hammer curling 100-pound dumbbells like the reincarnation of Atlas next to you. In fact, you may be pleased to hear that strength training doesn't have to involve any iron at all. Some of the best exercises you can do right in your own home, no equipment necessary. Your own body weight can serve as ample resistance for toning up those muscles, and these workouts are some of my personal favorites.

I prefer to work alternating muscle groups every other day. One day I'll do pushups and squats, the other day I'll do sit-ups and some form of back exercise. The reason for this is very simple. When muscles are broken down during exercise, there's a significant recovery period that is wise to commit to. Muscles take about 48 hours to fully rebuild themselves in preparation for their next trials. That means it's important that you take advantage of your workout every time you lift. Pump while the iron's hot. Lift to exhaustion in all your sets, and do sets until you can't finish any more reps. The number of reps is irrelevant, so long as you're doing your very best. Form is top priority, so check around on the Internet for how you should execute each move. One rep in proper form is worth more than five doing it incorrectly. Bad form is not only inefficient; it can result in outright injury.

It's better to work each muscle group for a set block of time. Don't do one set of sit-ups in the morning, one at lunch, and another before dinner. Exerting muscles after they've been broken down only hinders the recovery process and can squander the gains you've made. Do it hard, do it now, and get on with the rest of your day. When you've got a firm hold of the bodyweight exercises, start stepping it up. Put on a weight vest, or start hitting the bench at the gym. Whatever you do, keep to a regular routine. You'll find that your muscles start acting as tools, assisting your progression, rather than adversaries in chasing your gains.

    As with your diet, exercising is about trying new things and finding your particular cup of tea. If you prefer cycling to running, stick to cycling. If you like the leg press more than the dead lift, keep adding weights to that machine. Unless you're trying to impress the judges on Muscle Beach, sticking to just a few different exercises will keep you in pretty great shape. You don't ever have to leave the house if you prefer to keep to your abode, but the gym can be a great motivator in and of itself.

    Because let's face it, the gym can be a frightening environment. Men and women in optimal physical shape are still there busting their ass, lifting weights that make you question their superhuman abilities. Just remember, even the biggest, baddest mofo on the bench had to start somewhere. Most at the gym are concerned with his or her own vanity far more than taking the time to rag on a newcomer. In fact, you may even inspire others for showing up to better yourself. If you have any questions about the machines or strategies to maximize your results, fitness forums on the Internet or personal trainers at the gym are often more than willing to share their wisdom. You paid good money for your gym membership, so maximize the return out of your investment! I know it sounds cliché as fuck, but Rome wasn't built in a day, and neither was your body. That took 9 months. And in 9 months' time from today, you could put those old Romans to shame.

Engaging your muscles regularly isn't all about putting time in at the gym or running until you feel faint. Repeating these activities day in and day out can get rather mundane, and the last thing you want is to bore yourself with a routine. If you want to get in a good workout today but just can't stomach the gym, start doing some of those pesky chores you've been putting off. Take your car to the car wash and detail it by hand, inside and out. Scrub those tires and wheels until they shine like new. Wax on, wax off. Take a step back and gaze at what you've accomplished. Your car is going to be looking the best it has in a long time, plus you'll be feeling that sting of pride only known from the upkeep of one's possessions.

Mow the lawn, start a garden, or clean the roof gutters. Scrub the bathroom, sweep the kitchen, or vacuum the carpets. These activities take a little time and elbow grease, keeping you moving while distracting you from life's other nonsense. Furthermore, you never have to be droning along with the same thing more than once. Clean one area and clear out. Others take notice when you maintain a fresh looking castle, and they'll start to notice you too before long.

Even fans of video games are hopping on the fitness bandwagon. Gamers everywhere are setting up home gyms within distance of their PCs or consoles. What's more entertaining than a bike ride whilst shooting up zombies? How about a six mile walk as you're storming through the dungeons of Azeroth? Gaming exercise is a great tool in the sense that you can be fully immersed in another dimension while tuning out the struggles of physical work. Sure, there may be TV screens at the gym to provide you with a passive form of entertainment, but leaving this world entirely through games can push your mind even further away from the tasks you typically trudge over. Innovative technologies such as the *Omni* or *Oculus Rift* take it even one step further, inputting your physical movements into the game you're playing. Imagine taking a stroll through an alien landscape, blasting away Martians for hours as you ramp up your cardio. The future is now, so why not take advantage of it?

You could also take up a sport you've been meaning to get into. Recently, I reacquainted myself with the great game of golf, and it's now a favorite hobby of mine. It may seem like a rather leisurely game, but a golf swing works a lot of muscles in both the upper and lower body. If you want to kick it up a notch further, you could even ditch the cart in favor of walking the course, adding miles of hiking to your game. Try tennis or a game of squash with one of your friends, or shoot some basketballs around the court. Hell, even *bowling* counts as a sport. Make whatever activity you're doing a fun and productive part of your day. You won't be playing like Jordan Spieth or Stephen Curry on the first day out, but that's beside the point. The objective is to show up and play, not necessarily to play *well*. No one ever left the court or the gym after a couple of hours spouting off, "Gee, what a waste of time!"

Remember, exercise is *not* mandatory for weight loss, but it does accelerate things and can even be *fun*. Think of it like adding an extra shot of NOS to your metabolic engine. Nevertheless, I realize that no matter how much this guy or anyone else drills the thought of working out into your head, sometimes the motivation just isn't there. It's hard to exercise after a long day at work, or 14 years in a motorized cart. Hell, I prefer the couch to the bench any damned day of the week. And that's *fine*. The laws of thermodynamics are still a very real thing, and calorie deficits can be readily achieved through changing the diet alone.

11

Vitamins: Not Just for the Old Folks

Do you ever feel like the food you're eating is just not enough sometimes? Feeling hungry or lethargic throughout the day is not a pleasant experience, but for many it can be a straightforward fix. You know now about empty calories and how a high-calorie diet can still leave you starving at the end of the day. Well, one reason those hunger pangs are hanging over you like the Shanghai smog may be that you have an underlying vitamin deficiency.

Vitamins exist in all kinds of foods, and especially dense quantities can be found in fruits and vegetables. Heavily processed foods have a tendency to be stripped of these essential nutrients, leaving very little reason to eat them in their refined states. Thankfully, even when we choose not to eat a diverse range of foods in any given day, several over-the-counter supplements are available to help fulfill our bodies' wide-ranging needs.

It's always best to get vitamins and minerals from their

indigenous sources. For example, the natural calcium found in milk is much better for you than taking a synthesized calcium supplement. The human body is more able to recognize and uptake nutrients from natural origins, allowing you to reach your recommended daily levels in a more complete and sustainable way. Nonetheless, if you don't particularly care for a tall glass of milk or a Greek yogurt, any substitute you are willing to take is going to help you more than nothing at all.

Equally important as keeping yourself within an appropriate caloric range for your body, consistency in maintaining the accompanying levels of vitamins and minerals is key to your success. Don't expect to take one vitamin B12 pill a week and notice any tangible results in your health. Vitamins are depleted in our bloodstreams rather quickly, and some supplements may require you to take 2 or 3 capsules per day. Remember how Grandma kept telling you to take your vitamins? *Take your damn vitamins.*

There are so many different vitamins on the store shelves it can make your head spin. Some companies (i.e. The Vitamin Shoppe) have built entire empires by slinging every type of nutrient imaginable under one roof. Go to your local grocery store and you'll similarly find aisle after aisle full of supplements. So, you might ask, which ones should I take?

I'll start by pointing out the ones you don't need to take. Diet pills like Hydroxycut, Xenadrine, or whatever catchy new name they're slapping on the bottle these days do little to shed pounds. Most are little more than energy supplements, pumped full of the same kinds of ingredients you would find in a Red Bull or other energy drink. Sure, the model with the ripped abs on the box looks of the ideal human variety. But don't think for a second that they went from obese to swimsuit model by popping a couple of pills. Do you really believe those bodybuilders on the Bowflex commercials got huge on a machine that maxes out at 200 lbs.? Don't fall for these traps. There is no "revolutionary" weight loss solution on the shelves that makes it that simple.

What we can do, parlor tricks aside, is assist our bodies in operating at their peak metabolic efficiencies. When we suffer from vitamin deficiencies, our bodies have difficulty in processing newly eaten food and will resort to storing any excess fuel it sees as fat. That same vitamin deficiency will remain if you don't eat something to combat that lack of nutrient, leading the body to still crave more food. This cycle repeats *ad infinium*, further distancing us from the road to redemption.

As far as which vitamins I do recommend, let me preface this by saying once again that *I AM NOT A DOCTOR*. Especially if you are taking any prescription medications at all, make sure you check with a physician before adding supplements to your daily regimen. That said, I would say that some brands on the shelf are unequivocally better than others. Vitamins are not like prescription pills, and they are not subjected to the same strict guidelines mandated by the FDA.

One of the best indicators of quality is the price. Don't settle for the cheap stuff, especially when your health and wellbeing are at stake. Price alone is not enough to vouch for anything though, so what I like to do further is read reviews written by the people who have used these items. My go-to place for browsing most vitamins is Amazon.com, where many products already have hundreds of user ratings. Amazon has an entire category dedicated to vitamins and minerals, so you'll likely find anything and everything you need there.

To start, you're going to want to scope out a good multivitamin that appeals to you. This sets up the foundation to build upon, if nothing else. Multivitamins will help supplant a majority of your daily nutrient needs, and many ask that you only take one per day. Some of the more popular offerings are more synthetic than they ought to be (i.e. Centrum), but others are derived solely from whole foods, providing natural and sustainable health benefits. The latter mentioned ones will be those on the pricier side. Sort the long list of options by those with the highest review ratings and go from there. If 786 other people found one particular product helpful, there's a good chance you might as well.

A second supplement I would recommend you take is *fish oil*. Fish oil is known primarily for improving heart health, but there are some other distinct advantages as well. Fish oil stimulates muscular growth in the body by aiding in protein synthesis while decreasing protein breakdown. The omega-3s, DHA, and EPA found in fish oil also contribute to an enhanced immune system and a heightened sensitivity to insulin.

But wait, there's more! Call now and I'll double the offer (just pay separate Processing and Handling)! Another crucial benefit of fish oil is improved *brain health*. The mind is nothing without the body, and the brain struggles to be healthy when the body is anything but. Changing up the supplements you take (or adding some for the first time) can have an enormously positive impact on both. The fact that you're overweight in itself leads many health officials to seek out what may be an underlying cause, and depression is a prime suspect. People who are depressed are more susceptible to destructive behaviors, with binge eating among them. It's likely that all the garbage being shoveled into your body has generated a chemical imbalance in your mind, riddling your focus with thoughts of hopelessness and despair. But fear not, young Padawan. Many, if not all of these symptoms can be remedied by incorporating supplements (like fish oil) into a progressively healthier lifestyle.

Some other mood-livening supplements you might find helpful are St. John's Wort, 5-HTP, L-Theanine, and valerian root. If you can, try some of these options before pursuing the prescription medication route, as many SSRIs and other antidepressants are known to significantly promote weight *gain*. Again, *I AM NOT YOUR DOCTOR AND YOU SHOULD DO WHATEVER HE OR SHE SAYS*! Experiment with different vitamins and other supplements until you pinpoint your preferred cocktail. There's a good chance that what's right for you is different from what's right for me. Hang in there if you don't notice results right away. Try a regimen for a month, and then evaluate the progress of your mental state (or lack thereof). These new chemicals you're introducing to your body take time to undo the harmful mechanisms you've been firing on for years. It's a gradual change, but patience is a virtue.

Devoting your attention to mental wellbeing is going to be the game changer in fighting off an obesity relapse. You don't want to be eating Cheetos in front of a Jenny Craig six months from now with a cardboard sign, chanting "We Are the 95%!" There are many avenues by which to address depressive thoughts, but just as with weight loss, they require commitment and consistency to yield results. It's easy to stress all day long, with your mind racing a thousand miles per hour from the time you wake up until the time you crash. Just set aside a little stretch of "me" time, a period where you let your trifling worries drift away. Some people swear by meditation, even if takes just 15 minutes out of your morning. You may even enjoy Yoga, a symbiotic mesh of both exercise and meditation. Do a little something every day that makes you feel good on the inside. I think you'll find rather quickly that it translates to a fuller, more well-rounded you.

Okay, we got off on a little bit of a psychological tangent right there, so let's shift back now and end on the topic of physical health. If you're really looking to break out the big guns on fat shredding, there are a few natural aids that can be expeditiously helpful in giving your metabolism that much needed turbo charge. These products should be used in conjunction with some kind of workout plan, as the extra energy they give off may leave you jittery and anxious otherwise.

Off the top of my head, I can think of a few boosters such as green tea, caffeine, and capsaicin that may work for you. You can drink coffee or tea outright, but the active ingredients in these drinks can also be found in extracts. Caffeine works by elevating your heart rate, thereby increasing your overall energy output. Green tea has its fair share of caffeine as well, and for a bonus it is full of what's known as *catechins*, an antioxidant that particularly targets fat loss. Capsaicin you should already be very familiar with. It is the ingredient that gives peppers their potent spice. Jalapenos, habaneros, and other peppers don't just *taste* hot, either. They raise your internal body temperature, propelling your sweat glands into action. If your taste buds aren't much into the whole "temperature torture" thing, you can also find capsaicin in the vitamin aisle, usually in capsules of cayenne pepper.

I venture to say it would be in very poor taste if I didn't save my absolute favorite supplement for last, so let's end this chapter on a high note, shall we? In actuality, this last one I've got for you isn't so much a supplement as it is a time-honored panacea of a health tonic. The magical formula to which I am referring is none other than *apple cider vinegar*.

Antedating the chicken noodle soup and Sprite cure-all by well over a millennium, apple cider vinegar was an antidote fervently endorsed by the very father of medicine himself: Hippocrates. Medical professionals around the world today still swear by a creed bearing his name. You know the one that says, "Do no harm?" That's the Hippocratic Oath.

As far back as the year 400 BC, Hippocrates treated his patients with a mixture of apple cider vinegar and honey for a deluge of ailments. From the common cold to cancer, apple cider vinegar was thought by the doctor to cure, or at least treat, the symptoms afflicting the sufferers taken under his wing. Though the purported benefits in Hippocrates' time were based on individual observation at best, today it's astonishing how truly great a discovery apple cider vinegar has shown itself to be over the ages.

Search for apple cider vinegar online and see for yourself. The list of ailments it boasts to treat are lengthy, and quite frankly they read like the talking points of a snake oil salesman. Weight loss, diabetes, cancer, high blood pressure, high cholesterol, heartburn, teeth stains, sunburn, hair conditioning, wart removal, and acne removal are just a few bullet points I'm seeing on one page. You can even mix the vinegar with water and use it as an aftershave!

Okay, I get it. Quiet down. I can't hear myself over the bells of skepticism going off in your head. It sounds far too good to be true, right? Are these proponents really just pulling our leg here? Well, given that the men and women of the medical community have been treading in the ancestral footsteps of Hippocrates' for eons, there is little doubt they have been curious of his methods.

While the proverbial saying "an apple a day keeps the doctor away" is an often-touted claim, the vinegar, not the apple itself, may provide the most significant health benefits. All vinegars contain acetic acid, a compound that alters the pH levels within our bodies. A diet that is too acidic, which most westerners in the world survive today on, fosters an environment where health problems are more likely to manifest. Though an acid itself, the acetic acid in vinegar metabolizes within the body as a base, or alkaline substance. This raises the pH of the body to a more balanced level, neutralizing some of the potential threats (such as heartburn or ulcers) that lurk within a predominantly acidic environment.

As observed in clinical studies over the past decade, this property of alkalinity is also thought to be a factor in lowering blood glucose levels, suppressing appetite, and slowing fat accumulation, Though doctors disagree on the exact ingredient in apple cider vinegar makes it any healthier than another type of vinegar, most would suggest that the addition of some type of vinegar to the diet is largely beneficial. My high school Spanish teacher once shared with the class that he had been taking vinegar for the past 20 years, and he never once called in a single sick day. I've only been using ACV for about the past three or four years, but during this period, my overall health has never been better.

That's not to say there aren't some caveats, however. Undiluted vinegar is a rather caustic substance, and drinking it straight from the bottle can lend itself to the erosion of teeth enamel and the esophageal lining. What you want to do is measure out about 2 tablespoons of vinegar and mix it in a tall glass of water. Now, even this watered-down vinegar won't be the most palatable cocktail out there, so go ahead and mix in a dab of honey if the taste is still too strong.

Since I don't like the taste much either, I usually just chug the glassful in one go of it. I try to take at least twice of these drinks in a day, before mealtime. I do it beforehand for a couple of reasons. For one, I don't have to ruin the taste of a good meal by doing it afterwards. Also, the alkaline effects of vinegar are going to work against any spikes in blood sugar resulting from the food. Finally, the sheer hydration aspect of the drink alone is going to cause the stomach to feel fuller much earlier. The addition of two glasses of water in a daily ritual is near reason enough to take the plunge.

If I had to describe anything in this book as my "secret weapon", apple cider vinegar is it. My skin is smoother and less cracked, my hair is fuller and silkier, and it really gives off a powerhouse kick of energy immediately after taking it. But don't just take my cultist's appreciation at face value. Whether it's merely a tool of folk medicine or a bona fide fat flayer, I'd say vinegar is at least an avenue worth checking out. Read some of the reviews on Amazon, and see how other people's experiences relate to you. Most habitual imbibers recommend Bragg's brand products, as they're organic and contain all the unfiltered nutrients of raw apples.

Lastly, do some casual research online and see what other dietary supplements you think might help your cause. There's no such thing as a magical fat-burning pill, but a combination of the products I've listed here and others do help facilitate a more advantageous bodily ecosystem. Picture it as if you're switching out your old computer at the office. You still have to get the report done by Friday, but now you're much less likely to have it crash and be forced to start all over again.

12

The Anarchist's Diet

ATTENTION: *The extreme weight loss methods I'm about to mention here are potentially very hazardous to your health and may even cause your untimely death. Take extreme precaution before you even think about trying any of these!*

And now, ladies and gentlemen, we descend deep into the annals of the diet dark web. You've reached the point of no return, and you're safety is no longer guaranteed (not that it was to begin with). While I'm a firm believer that diet and exercise is the best long-term approach to health, you may simply not be willing to delay the gratification of possessing a slim figure. If you're prepared to forego the commitment aspect of this whole "diet thing" and aren't perturbed by the risk of serious consequences, this section's for you.

Others have gambled their lives on these shortcuts, because *they work*. At least in the short term, they do. You'll likely see enormous returns in the outset, and you may even start to believe that your present choices are laying the groundwork for a sustainable lifestyle. They are not. I came to the conclusion that you should at least know the wagers being placed with these timesavers before impetuously going out and ruining your life.

Many of the tricks you've doubtlessly heard before or maybe have even tried already, so we'll do a quick roundup of the mega trends. Perhaps the safest way to guarantee significant amounts of weight loss is to go under the knife of a bariatric surgeon. Roux-en-Y gastric bypass surgery, colloquially known as "stomach stapling", remains the most popular option available to people who are at least 100 lbs overweight. You may have seen the TLC show "My 600LB Life", where quarter-ton patients are rolled into operating rooms for this quick escape from morbidity.

In case you're not aware of what's exactly involved with such an operation, allow me to clue you in on the highlights. First off, a nice long incision (or several smaller ones in laparoscopic) is cut right down the center of your abdomen, permitting access to your insides. Then, the doctor lops off your stomach right near the top, and the two cut pieces get stapled shut. Moving below the stomach, your small intestine is severed a ways down and stitched together with the upper, walnut-sized stomach portion (still clinging to the lower esophagus). But wait, there's more. The bulky lower stomach provides vital acids that aid in digestion, so the part of the small intestine still connected to the lower stomach is reattached to the raised portion of the small intestine further down the chain. This creates the "Y" junction of the Roux-en-Y procedure (Roux is the doctor it's named after), permitting stomach juices to flow down and break up foods. Finally, after all this butchery, the surgeon often elects to just rip out your gall bladder, as gallstones begin to appear with greater frequency in people who lose rapid amounts of weight.

If that sounds like more hacking than you're willing to put up with, the *adjustable gastric band* (or lap-band, as it were) may offer a better "fit" for you. In this procedure, surgeons attach a constricting circular band around the upper portion of the stomach, isolating a small pouch that helps you feel fuller faster. Requiring far less sewing and stitching, the lap-band offers a friendlier alternative to the easily squeamish. Though this band has the potential to slip, and must be routinely adjusted to work in its optimal capacity, many patients report similar successes in total weight lost compared to gastric bypass. It has the added advantage of being a reversible operation, too.

Bypass patients have the advantage of losing weight

faster initially, but a greater percentage will run into complications following surgery. Though mortality rates are relatively minute (0.3% of patients after 90 days), up to 14.5% will suffer anomalies that may require more surgery to fix. Other than the normal risks associated with abdominal surgery (infection, hemorrhaging, hernia, bowel obstruction), ulcers may form, stomach acid could leak, and scarring resulting from the operation might block food from passing through the new plumbing. Also, the post-operation diet is such a restrictive and radical change that patients often cause more problems on their own. Stretching the stomach by not adhering to proper portion control could even render the operation fruitless.

 Whichever way you go, chances are you're going to end up wanting more surgeries later on. Though you may lose 250 lbs. in a year's time, your skin will not be able to keep up the pace, leaving drapes of your rind hanging in every undesirable region. You may find that the fat lost has been grossly disproportional in some areas, and liposuction may be your only option to combat it. These subsequent nips and tucks will escalate the costs sizably, as cosmetic procedures are generally not covered by your health insurance. But could you live with yourself if you went through all the trouble of gastric bypass just to have arms that look like elephant ears? I guess the free wingsuit wouldn't be so bad.

Moving on from the safety and comfort of physician-supervised weight loss, let's go over some of the ways in which we can self-induce similar outcomes. This would be the allegorical final step off the continental shelf of rationality.

We can obviously choose to not eat at all (anorexia), which would seem like a rather elementary fix. Too much food = fat, no food = awesome! Indeed, this would seem to be the very best course of action, except for the equally elementary fact that *starvation* is inevitable.

When food is scarce, the body is quick to recognize this imminent threat and enters what is known as a state of *ketosis*, the so-called "starvation mode" you hear about. In ketosis, the body begins to devour itself of fat stores for fuel, which (you guessed it) means you start losing weight. People who follow a *ketogenic diet* or other low-carb diet (like Atkins) purposefully activate this survival response to shed pounds, because the body eats consumed fat at an accelerated pace. With anorexia, you're not even getting any of the nutritional benefits provided by one of these fat-filled diets, leading to full-on *malnutrition*. This can cause any number of diseases and ailments that a vitamin or mineral deficiency might contribute to. Everybody quits anorexia one way or another. If you choose to live and start eating normally again, ketosis is going to store every last carbohydrate back on your body as fat. That's part of the reason why crash dieters typically gain back even more than what they initially lose.

As long as we're talking about anorexia, we might as well drag her bastardized cousin *bulimia* right into the mix. Binging and purging can be just as harmful as anorexia, though you may be able to get away with it for a longer period of time. Bulimia is the fun eating disorder, because you can indulge incessantly on whatever food you like. Eat that entire cake or tray of brownies if you wish. *It ain't going to the hips, but back through your lips!*

Immediately following your gluttonous binge, finding a way to evacuate the revolting contents becomes the preeminent imperative. Self-induced vomiting remains the most popular choice, with many engaging the gag reflex with ipecac syrup (used for poison control) or simply jamming a finger down the pie hole. Some find solace ingesting large quantities of laxatives, shooting the food through the intestines before the body ever has a chance to recognize they ate it. The least effective way is to take diuretics, so-called "water pills" that flush retained water from the system. Each of these methods can harm the body immensely, with problems ranging from dehydration to a damaged gastrointestinal tract or heart problems. However, you probably won't *die* as a result of bulimia. Whether you're upchucking or down-chucking, the body will still find a way to grab a portion of those calories from the food. You might even *gain* weight as a bulimic if you binge too much.

Drug abuse, both legal and illegal, is another beautifully dangerous weapon in the extreme dieters' arsenal. Exploiting drugs to one's advantage can be as easy as failing to take enough insulin for a diabetic, leaving blood sugar at dangerously high (but carb indigestible) levels. People who are prescribed stimulating drugs, like Ritalin for Attention Deficit Disorder, may find their drugs are better suited for exercise than studying for a calculus exam.

MDMA, cocaine, and methamphetamine invigorate their users with hours upon hours of energy. You may have seen people passing around mollies at a music rave, fueling their long night of dancing and pumping of the fists. Rob Ford's not only famous for being the crack-smoking mayor of Toronto, but perhaps for also being the world's *fattest* crack head. Even more benign substances like marijuana increase the heart rates of its users. Weed's analgesic effects just might breach the mental barrier of exercise too, turning a workout from a nightmarish affair into a delightful experience.

Then there are the performance-enhancing drugs. Steroids, human growth hormone, and even deer antlers are glamorized in the news for their athlete contract-killing potential. Most of us are not regularly subjected to such drug evaluations, though, enabling their uninhibited use in gyms across the globe. Though not necessarily intended for weight loss, these drugs help build mountains of calorie-hungry muscle, essentially meeting the same ends. Some substances are legal while others are not, but most are known to significantly strengthen muscular ability well beyond what humans are normally capable of. If you are especially weak to start with, steroids might give you enough of a confidence kick to get back in the gym. Be careful of who you get your supply from, though. Other than the occasional fit of 'roid rage you might encounter, be on the lookout for tainted drugs. And never share needles with your bench spotter. Mad gains aren't worth the side of HIV, I'm positive.

Sticking with the theme here, it wouldn't be fair if I didn't save the deadliest substance for last. If you're looking for a special something that helps you lose weight while guaranteeing to kill you, tobacco is it. Cigarettes have been a vice of slender people for ages. Nicotine is a well-known stimulant and appetite suppressant, two properties of which I can personally attest to. As a regular smoker, I was far likelier to skip an afternoon snack in favor of a few drags off a coughing nail. I could often skip a full meal entirely, or at least delay eating for a few hours if need be. We're all aware of the immensely destructive consequences of smoking long term, and I don't recommend at all that you go down to the 7/11 and pick up a carton of Newports right this minute. However, I reason that I would rather live 10 years less as a thinner person than whale about for an extra decade. Can you stay thin without cigarettes? Absolutely. Is it better to step outside for a cig than make a turn for the snack drawer? That's a question you'll have to answer for yourself.

It's not my intention to help you devolve into a pill-popping animal or push you to go under the knife. My hope instead is that you take to heart some of these options that others before you have tried, and do whatever you can to avoid stumbling from an addiction to food into another snare of dependency. You may be able to "fake it until you make it" with some of these unconventional tactics, but defrauding your body of the dedication and willpower it deserves will only get you so far in life.

13

Ascension

I set about writing this award-winning masterpiece nearly two years ago, yet as I neared the finish line I found myself overcome several times with a deep sense of writer's block. I felt I had expressed what needed to be said. But there was a missing element, a piece of the puzzle that had yet to be conjoined to a seemingly complete image.

Then it dawned on me. What was lacking was a definitive conclusion to my epic tale of woes and wonderment. Sure, I can share with you the circumstances I found myself in and the choices I made that led to my unsatisfactory condition. I can expound upon the methods of madness I employed to unearth myself from those torturous binds of permanence. What I didn't have two years ago was a conclusion to the story, a paradigm shift that could show how losing weight has made truly catalyzing change possible in my life. Now, I can share with you just how radical that change can be.

About two and a half years ago, I walked into an office that I had never thought I would walk into it my entire life. For an obese man, that of course was a military recruiter's office. It was a hot July day in Arizona, and I had no other particularly pressing business going on that day, so I decide to go for it. I walked into the office like any unknown, and I told them and I wanted to be a pilot. He said, "No, son, you want to be a navigator!" So, I signed up to be a navigator.

Unfortunately, it takes a lot more these days to become an officer in the United States military then running into the office waving your college degree around. No, today the application process is so long you can finish your master's degree in the process (which is exactly what I did). I went out to Luke Air Force Base to take the equivalent of the enlisted ASVAB test, as well as the TBAS (another test that gauges your ability to fly). I also went about filling out the Bible's worth of paperwork attached to a military officers application, several articles of which I had to submit multiple times because they were lost in the system or somehow incorrect. I also had to submit several affidavits concerning my felonious past, and why I would never commit such unspeakable offenses going forward. So, I completed the test (which I happened to do very well on), I submitted all my paperwork, and then I got a phone call shortly afterwards saying that the Air Force was suspending recruitment indefinitely.

I was told to keep my applications current in the event that they did reopen their slots, so, not having anything better to do, I did. And, through the persistence I had over the next couple of years, my patience and the support of my friends and family paid off. I received a call on another hot Arizona day in July in 2015 and my recruiter shared with me the good news that I was to begin Officer Training School on October 6th. It was the news that many people, including myself, had begun to think would never come. Sequestration has severely limited amount of new officers and enlisted personnel inducted into the armed services, and at that time less than 20% of applicants where approved. But when they told me long ago that 95% of dieters are unsuccessful, I knew this endeavor would be a breeze.

So, I did what any sane man would do , and I moved out of the house , sold most of my belongings , left my dog, and drove across the country to start a new job . I suppose that it qualifies as an adventure more than a job, really. The truth of the matter is: I didn't know what I was getting myself into. I still don't, to a large extent.

I made it through the nine week course at Maxwell Air Force Base in Montgomery, Alabama, and now I'm currently stationed at Pensacola Naval Air Station awaiting training as a combat systems officer, or CSO. You know Goose, from *Top*

Gun? Yeah, that's one of the jobs I could be doing soon. I must say that it has been a truly stellar experience thus far, and I feel that this life course I chose has contributed significantly to my personal growth.

This is the first time that I've been away from family for an extended period of time, and I wasn't too sure I'd be able to handle it. With that said, my experience with the Air Force up to this point has been nothing short of extraordinary. The people around me are nothing short of the finest, and I've been given the chance to do many things that are simply not possible in the civilian realm. I went through Initial Flight Training in Pueblo, Colorado, and for my checkride I flew around a Major in a tiny little plane not even the size of a Cessna. I doubt that I'll have the opportunity to say that I piloted around a field grade officer for the rest of my career. I'll be taking the backseat from here on out. Never would I ever have thought I would be traversing the snowy wildness of Washington for SERE training, either.

As an aside, I must say that being a casual lieutenant is perhaps the best paying gig on planet Earth. You see, as I'm waiting the undergraduate CSO training to start, I am on what's known as "casual status." What that means is I have to show up at 7:45 in the morning, 5 days a week, to what's called muster. At muster, there's a lieutenant there with bulletins that apply to the day's business, which can range anywhere from paperwork that needs to be done to volunteer opportunities in the local area. What that means personally is that I'm *usually* done for the day by around 8 o'clock in the morning. It often takes me longer to get dressed in fatigues than for the announcements to be read. From then on, I'm free to do pretty much whatever I please for the day. I can go play golf on the base course, I can go to the mall, or I can go to the beach. Then I wake up the next morning and do it all again. Except we have mandatory PT three days a week. On those days, I'll be working straight through the late hour of nine in the morning. I'm assured by my peers in training ahead of me and higher authority that this paradise on earth is most assuredly short-lived.

I am happy when I am working, though. I realize that the work I'm doing is fulfilling a cause far greater than my own, whatever that may be. They've given me access to a fully furnished, one-bedroom apartment (utilities paid for), and they push on me thousands of dollars a month to learn how to fly airplanes. I think I made the right choice. The beaches here are the pearliest of white, and the sand is so fine that it squeaks between your toes. The people are warm and welcoming, and the alcohol is cold and plentiful. Many days I wake up and I find myself wondering if I'm merely traversing a dream, a projection of a life that is not my own. That's how wonderful this moment in for me truly is. Eternally grateful does not even begin to describe how appreciative I am for this opportunity. And now is only the beginning for me. The future holds nothing but the promise of great things to come.

Final Thoughts

What's life like at the end of the tunnel? Is a mere change in my appearance really worth all the time, effort, and hardship? Is it even possible for me? Personally, I have to respond with an emphatic, unequivocal, "Yes!" You know it too, or else why the hell have you kept reading all this time? You know the phrase "beauty is only skin deep." Well, you probably also know that if you're ugly on the outside, most people won't even give you the time of day to prove your inner worth. Why would I pick the bruised apple over the shiny one, even if the good-looking one were rotten to the core? It's because first impressions count for a lot in this life. Appearance *is* reality.

Are you lazy, or worse yet, dumb? I know I sure as hell was, but not anymore! Whip that body into shape and revel in how hard working and kept together others perceive you as. *It's nothing short of a miracle, I tell ya!* A fat body is almost assuredly a sign that your IQ is 20 points lower than anyone else in the room, not to mention you've never lifted a finger a day in your life. You could be the most toiling genius out there right now, and no one would take your word for it. At first glance, I know I sure as hell wouldn't.

It may be the fact that eating chicken and waffles for breakfast on a regular basis is just *not* an intelligent thing to do. Plus, you're lazy because you didn't at least work the Aunt Jemima off by bedtime. It's likely a combination of both forces, which is exactly how the masses will piece it together at a cursory glance.

The simple act of going outside the house should be much easier for the slimmer you. Not worrying about people judging your every move is an incredibly relieving change of pace. You can start to mill about the world like a normal human being for once, rather than a pariah to mock and scorn. Some people in your life will even look up to you for guidance, which is precisely why I wanted to write this book. If you are, one day, blessed with the gift of better health, it's important that you give back and share your experiences with the people you love. Though they may be resistant to your advice, and keep on meandering through an existence clouded by denial and self-harm, making yourself available for a person in the throws of a food addiction can make all the difference in the world. Be that inspiration. *If I can do it, so can you!*

Becoming a role model in your own right keeps that

fire of motivation lit beneath yourself. The Battle of the Bulge is only the opening stages of your personal War on Obesity. The struggle with weight loss is lifelong campaign. 20 years (or even two years) from now, I might gain every last ounce of what I lost back. The longer you keep it off, though, the longer you should expect to see continued success. A battle-hardened dieter is wary of the traps and pitfalls littering his or her road ahead, and he or she can plan accordingly.

In the broader sense, my health has immeasurable improved since I shed the excess fat, and I'm positive yours will too. It wasn't uncommon for me to come down with bronchitis for several weeks every winter, hacking and coughing well into the night. Cold spells or strep throat incapacitated me for several months of my childhood years. Severe indigestion reared its ugly head almost every time I ate, especially if I indulged myself out at a restaurant. Pepto Bismol was my after-dinner mint. Random joint pain or abdominal pain could show up at any time for no apparent reason at all. Hell, I even faked illness on occasion just to avoid having to go to school, but that ties in with a fear of getting bullied more than anything.

Have you ever been sick for so long that you forgot what feeling well was like? That's how I equate my obese self to now. I'm amazed at just how much better in general I feel after cutting that fat tumor out. Sure, after a couple of years, I've become accustomed to it. But looking back now, I can't remember the last time I was couch-locked due to an illness. I've been imbibed with the youthful sense of immortality so many older folks warn our generation about.

The frequency of smiles, ass grabbings, and flirtatious playings of the hair in my general direction has increased dramatically, and that's something you too have to look forward to. Life as a whole, I must say, is definitely headed in the right direction. Who knows? Maybe this book right here will launch my career as a bestselling, Pulitzer Prize winning author! Probably not, but it never hurts to dream.

I could whip up a couple of more anecdotes about how life in the present is nothing but unicorns and rose petals, but that would be wholly disingenuous. If you think weight loss is going to solve all of the problems you have today, be mindful that this is far from the case. Shedding pounds is not going to wondrously confer onto you the power of a magnetic personality or land you that high paying job. If people think of you as a miserable cunt today, that opinion is not going to change in the course of a few months, or a few inches off your waistline. What will change, though, is the volume of opportunities *you* have to be cordial.

If you've been overweight or obese for any length of time, you know just how cruel another human being can be. Whether spoken "in jest" or as a direct insult, their hurtful words and insinuations can condition you over time not just to hate yourself, but nearly everyone around you. This prejudice of revulsion takes awhile to get over, and I still find myself reluctant at times to crack a smile at a stranger. The fact is that, when you lose the pounds, people will find you automatically more approachable and likable. But for years I've witnessed the duality of man, so oftentimes it's difficult for me to respond amicably to this newfound kindness of others without first ruminating on their motives.

I find, however, that it's imperative to keep a positive attitude, despite how fake or facetious I know that person I'm talking to really be. Hate only cedes power back into the hands of the hector that made your life hell. I've said it before, but the sweetest revenge is a life well lived, and looking good is a part of that. The negative, unsolicited comments about your appearance or way of life are never going to end, but the accomplishment of keeping off the weight will help fortify your self-image in shrugging off the cynics. *Haters gonna hate*.

Third-party opinions are invalid, so long as the most important appraiser (you) voids their merit. Thin and athletic people get every bit as self-conscious of their physiques as the fatties. There are many days where I look in the mirror and see my old, morbidly obese self, locking eyes with me. Like it or not, remnants of memories past can and will surface to the forefront. That's life. Just as you remember in bed how awkward you were in that one conversation you had eight years ago, there will be times when you revisit your grotesque existence and feel down about it.

If there's one thing I can share with you today that can help boost your self-esteem, it's to realize that most human beings are largely engrossed with themselves. Though you may appear to be the center of the known universe, everyone else is at the heart of his or her own. Most people don't give a damn about your imperfections (or accomplishments, for that matter), and the ones who do are typically masking their own flaws by accentuating yours. Don't fret and become your own harshest critic, focusing singularly on the negative, because it benefits absolutely *no one*. Wear your stretch marks and saggy skin with pride, for they are the battle scars of a war for which *you* wrote the history books. Believe that your potential self is still greater than the kinetic, and you will reap the fortunes of prosperity.

I will leave you now to pursue the destiny that you alone were born to forge. I have illuminated the aisle to reinvention, and by passing the torch, I have served the usefulness of my purpose. Will you save yourself from the hell you created of this earth, or will you succumb to the vast and prodigious forces of evil? Only the sands of time will tell.

Banish me now to the catacombs of your bookshelf, and begin anew. I bid you good day, and good luck.

Made in United States
North Haven, CT
24 February 2023